Sports Medicine:

Health Care for Young Athletes

Second Edition

Author: Committee on Sports Medicine and Fitness
American Academy of Pediatrics

Paul G. Dyment, MD, Editor

American Academy of Pediatrics
141 Northwest Point Blvd
PO Box 927
Elk Grove Village, IL 60009-0927

COMMITTEE ON SPORTS MEDICINE AND FITNESS 1985-1991

Library of Congress Catalog Card No. 82-073444

ISBN No. 0-910761-28-0

Quantity prices on request. Address all inquiries to:
American Academy of Pediatrics
141 Northwest Point Boulevard, PO Box 927
Elk Grove Village, Illinois 60009-0927

ACKNOWLEDGMENTS

The Committee gratefully acknowledges the help of Crystal Milazzo, project manager with the Division of Child and Adolescent Health, for supervising the preparation of this manual, and the following individuals who contributed the initial drafts of chapters:

Oded Bar-Or, MD, FAAP,
   McMaster University, Hamilton, Ontario, Canada
Paul G. Dyment, MD, FAAP,
   Maine Medical Center, Portland, ME
Barry Goldberg, MD, FAAP,
   Yale University, New Haven, CT
Suzanne B. Haefele, MD, FAAP,
   Rock Hill, SC
Richard Malacrea, ATC,
   Princeton University, Princeton, NJ
James H. Moller, MD, FAAP,
   University of Minnesota, Minneapolis, MN
John J. Murray, MD, FAAP,
   Burlington, VT
Michael A. Nelson, MD, FAAP,
   Albuquerque, NM
David M. Orenstein, MD, FAAP,
   University of Pittsburgh, Pittsburgh, PA
Arthur M. Pappas, MD, FAAP,
   University of Massachusetts, Worchester, MA
William L. Risser, MD, FAAP,
   University of Texas, Houston, TX

INTRODUCTION: SPORTS MEDICINE AND PEDIATRICIANS

The first edition of *Sports Medicine: Health Care for Young Athletes* was published in 1983, and it quickly found a large audience. It answered the need to have in one place a body of knowledge concerning sports medicine necessary for the primary care physician. The field of sports medicine is rapidly changing, and this edition has been completely rewritten, chapters added and deleted, and our hope is that it reflects an office-practice perspective.

Pediatricians are accustomed to adapting to advances in the health sciences and to at least coping with social changes. The numerous innovations in immunizations and medical technology, a heightened watchfulness for evidence of child abuse, concerns about preventing childhood injuries and poisonings, and vigilance for indications of substance abuse all indicate new directions in pediatrics. Having assimilated these and other developments in child health care into their practices, many pediatricians are now becoming increasingly involved in sports medicine, an area traditionally considered the preserve of orthopedic surgeons. However, the field of sports medicine encompasses far more than the management of athletic trauma, and, even if it were restricted to managing injuries, most of them can be successfully treated by primary care physicians.

Our concept of the expanded role for pediatricians interested in sports medicine requires that they be familiar with the principles of physical fitness, exercise physiology, the prevention of athletic injuries, the psychology of youth, effective coaching techniques, and stress management. The practitioner should also act as an advocate for youth sports, exerting influence on school districts to ensure that physical education classes emphasize physical fitness and lifetime sports rather than team sports, which, although they have many positive features such as the development of character, will not be played by the participants once they begin their adult lives.

Our nation appears to have an increasing interest in physical fitness, vigorous recreation, and competitive sports. All persons, particularly youth, enjoy and need competition for personal satisfaction, status, and social acceptance. Most children are eager to test their bodies and skills against their peers. The child who wonders "Can I work that swing?" soon thinks, "How high can I swing?" and, eventually, "I think I can swing higher than John and Mary." Older children frequently have their best competitive experiences in sports activities.

More than 6 million boys and girls are taking part in competitive sports in high schools, and nearly 20 million more are engaged in out-of-school recreational and competitive sports, so-called "community sports." The latter are far less likely than high schools to have an acceptable program of health care supervision that will prevent injuries. For most physicians the sports physical examination is their only contact with sports medicine. What happens between the physician's approval to play and the patient's first injury or withdrawal from sports is usually not known by the physician.

The "sports physical" (better called a preparticipation examination) is not simply a procedure to separate the fit from the unfit. The wide variety of sports and the different physical requirements for contact sports, endurance sports, and those that emphasize skill allow physicians to recommend at least some kind of sport for nearly everyone, even those with impaired health or who are below par in their physical fitness, size, or maturation. Exclusion from physical activities, especially sports activities, can be detrimental to the boy or girl who is naturally alert, sociable, and competitive. By counseling about choices in sports and encouraging prompt treatment of injuries and health problems, a physician can help a young athlete have a worthwhile and maturing sports experience. Complete exclusion from sports activities can usually be avoided by having the physician act as the athlete's advocate and avoiding a hasty decision preventing all athletic activities.

Good health is not the only factor to be considered for safe participation in sports. Physical conditioning–for endurance, strength, agility, flexibility, body composition (ie, degree of fat), and acclimatization to heat and humidity–is also essential for a young athlete's performance and safety. Physicians need to know enough about physical conditioning procedures to evaluate specific needs for different sports and, ideally, to be prepared to give practical advice about methods for conditioning. Counseling the young athlete about nutrition, injury prevention, and the relative risks of injury in the different sports may need to be discussed with the athletes and their parents.

Most acute injuries in sports can be managed competently by pediatricians. One study showed that 2% of all office visits to one pediatric practice (a health maintenance organization) were for recreational injuries. Although fractures and severe sprains generally lie in the province of the orthopedic surgeon, most other injuries–contusions, strains, or mild sprains–can be managed quite successfully by a pediatrician.

Many physicians serve as team physicians for team sports. If they take this task seriously, they will be involved in educating the athletes and coaches on nutrition, pregame meals, injury prevention, and rehabilitation after injury as well as being on hand for acute injuries during games.

This volume attempts to provide that information necessary to make the pediatrician knowledgeable in what could be called "primary-care sports medicine." We hope that physicians who read this book will incorporate sports medicine into their child health-care practices.

Paul G. Dyment, MD, FAAP
Editor

CONTENTS

Chapter 8
Steroids

Chapter 9
Physical Fitness

Chapter 13
The Team Physician

Chapter 14
Rehabilitation

Chapter 15
The Athletic Trainer

Chapter 16
Initial Management of Minor Soft-Tissue Trauma

Chapter 17
Fractures and Dislocations

Chapter 18
Acute Knee Injuries

Chapter 19
Head and Neck Injuries

Chapter 20
Chronic Health Problems

LIST OF TABLES

LIST OF FIGURES

CHAPTER 1

ANTICIPATORY GUIDANCE
ABOUT PHYSICAL ACTIVITY

We live at a time when children are becoming more sedentary. Just as mechanization is decreasing the need for adults to be active in accomplishing work, school systems are decreasing the amount of physical activity for children in deference to more instructional time. Children spend enormous amounts of time watching television, playing computer games, and performing other sedentary activities. Free play time is decreasing, related in part to the inability of families with two working parents or single parents to supervise physical activities. In spite of controversies regarding appropriateness of the testing, national fitness studies consistently show America's children lagging behind those of other societies.[1]

The role of the physician in providing anticipatory guidance as well as responding to family inquiries regarding sports and exercise is vital. From the time a child is born, issues surrounding physical activity and exercise become important. Parents are bombarded by commercial ventures extolling the virtues of structured exercise plans. Parents will greatly appreciate the physician who has recommendations for exercise and sports available on a regular basis during health maintenance visits.

Table 1 lists subjects that the responsible primary care physician should discuss with parents, children, and young adults during health maintenance visits.

Infants

The infant's natural curiosity and interaction with other children and adults will adequately stimulate motor activity and develop proprioceptive skills.[2] There is no evidence to show that commercial products or organized exercise programs offer any advantage to babies. Throughout these first few months of life normal play with a child will ensure the full development of motor skills for which a child has been genetically endowed.

Although infants usually hold their breath instinctively when immersed, they continue to swallow water. The swallowed water may be absorbed into the bloodstream in quantities great enough to produce hyponatremia, which can lead to seizures several hours *after* the swimming class. Giardia may be transmitted through ingestion of contaminated pool water. Infants before age 3 or 4 months should not participate in swimming programs. As the infant becomes more mobile around 6 to 9 months of age, parents need to be cautioned to seal off standing water in pools, bathtubs, or ditches, and never to leave the child unattended.

Toddlers and Preschoolers

Parents of toddlers should be encouraged to participate with their children in active games such as "hide and go seek." Children's television watching time should be limited to no more than one hour a day, even for good programming. By age 3 the child should have regular opportunities to engage in active play with groups of several children through either preschool centers, day care, church groups, or neighborhood play groups. These experiences should emphasize free play and active play rather than structured play designed by adults. Family outings for walks and exploratory trips offer parents the opportunity to be good role models.

It is important again to emphasize water safety for the preschool child. Children of this age cannot ever be considered water safe.

School-Aged Children

Parents and school-aged children should be introduced to the concepts of fitness and its relationship to mental well-being, learning skills, and subsequent cardiovascular health. Studies in France and Canada seem to indicate that children who participate in additional physical activity in the school curriculum experience no delays in educational progress and may have enhanced "tools of intelligence" (ie, attentiveness) and perform better academically than students in the average curriculum. These findings occurred in spite of spending one third less time on academic study in preference to exercise and sports.[3,4] School boards should be encouraged to provide daily physical education classes. If school systems will not increase physical activity time, parents should encourage their children to stay active in their home lives. The long-term advantage cardiovascularly in people who continue active life styles is well known. However, overzealous pressure to participate in sports or endurance activities may result in burnout.

By the time their children are 6 years of age, parents should be encouraged to provide them with swimming instruction.

At approximately 6 to 8 years of age, children are attracted to community youth sports. It has been estimated that 75% of children participate in youth sport programs. By the time they reach high school, the number of children participating in organized sports programs dwindles to approximately 20%. Why do all these children drop out of organized sports?

Many experts postulate that there is too much emphasis in formal sports programs on the elite athlete and on winning. When attention is focused on elite athletes, all but the outstanding players are likely to become discouraged and drop out of organized sports. Parents need to be counseled regarding the readiness of their children to participate in team sports (ie, what are their social and physical maturation skills?) and to select programs and coaches whose primary interest in the sport is for the children to have FUN.

Strength training with weights can be of benefit to prepubertal children.[5] Fixed weights or Nautilus-type equipment are preferable. When strength training, children should always have adult supervision. If free weights are used, an adult "spotter" should participate to ensure against injury from falling barbells. Weight lifting (attempting to lift as much as one can) serves no useful purpose and is more likely than strength training to produce injuries.

In the active child, aerobic exercise is of limited benefit before puberty, although it may raise aerobic capacity by as much as 15%.[6] The sedentary obese child will benefit the most from increased aerobic activity provided in a structured format. Left to their own devices, obese children in interactive play still will be relatively inactive. When an obese child says he is active in sports, always ask more questions, or you may never find out that when he plays soccer he is always the goalie.

As they reach middle childhood, youngsters become more adventuresome in their activities. There is more risk taking. Parents and children should be counseled regarding safety involving such activities as bicycling and skateboarding, including the necessity of wearing a safety helmet and protective padding. They should avoid the use of any type of trampoline because of the risk of catastrophic spinal cord injury.

Adolescents

The physician should counsel the teen-ager more intensely regarding the benefits of exercise and fitness. Athletic conditioning such as weight control, necessity of adequate fluid intake during exercise, and strength and endurance training, addressed elsewhere in the text, should be discussed.

Safety rules regarding protective equipment such as helmets for bicycle riding, horseback riding, or off-road vehicles should be emphasized. Risk taking should be discouraged. Adolescents should be discouraged from using inherently dangerous vehicles such as motor bikes, motorcycles, and all-terrain vehicles.

For those adolescents not involved in regular organized sports activities, the benefits of regular exercise and its impact on fitness should be discussed. Some adolescents appear to need the benefits provided by highly competitive contact or collision sports. However, many parents and adolescents have little knowledge regarding the fitness value of many sports and exercise programs. Everyone should be aware of which sports contribute the most to cardiorespiratory endurance (Table 2).

Common Questions

1. *At what age should a child begin playing a team sport?*
The best age for each child is determined by his or her own pattern of development and expressed interest. Children begin at about age 6 to compare themselves with others in both skills and abilities and can play team sports. Most children can begin to play collision sports by the time they are 8 to 10 years old. Late-maturing adolescents should delay entry into collision sports against physically mature opponents.

The real question should be: Does the child want to participate in the team sport or do the parents want it? Some clues to the child's interest are pride in wearing a uniform, collecting sports items, or talking about sports.

Sports development is the same as other areas of the child's development; the more a child is pushed, the less likely are successes and the more he or she will resist. Thus, premature involvement may lead to early withdrawal because of boredom, pressure, or failure.

2. *Should I let my child quit a team?*
Before a parent reacts to a child's declaration that he or she wants to quit, it is necessary to gather the facts. The first step is to talk to the child. Although commitment to play a team sport should not be taken lightly, there are acceptable reasons to allow a child to withdraw. Valid reasons include (1) the coach is abusive and lacks skills to coach the child, and (2) the child is experiencing stress-related symptoms such as vomiting, headaches, or depression. No benefit is derived from playing under these circumstances, and continued participation may only result in the occurrence of more problems.

3. *How can a child with disabilities participate in sports activities?*
Very few disabilities preclude participation in all sports. Sports involvement offers psychologic and physical benefits for young people who have health-related handicaps. Some disabled adolescents desire to participate in sports activities that parents and physicians feel are inappropriate for them. In such instances, unless the activity would endanger the adolescent (eg, a hemophiliac playing football), he or she should make the final decision. The physician's responsibility is to

assess the handicap, arrange for consultation when necessary, recommend a physical fitness program, and alert the parents and adolescent to the pros and cons of participation. If the handicapped adolescent decides to participate, the parents and physician should be sure that appropriate equipment is available and used (eg, an athlete with only one good eye should use protective glasses).

4. *Should a child having trouble with academic work be allowed to participate in sports activities?*

There is no simple answer to this question. The child having difficulty in the classroom still needs the benefit of exercise, competition, and a sense of accomplishment. Sports activities may be an important means of success for a young person who is not experiencing success in the classroom. In some cases, the family and school may decide that the child is not studying hard enough. In this situation it is reasonable to make sports involvement dependent upon achieving better grades.

5. *Should boys and girls play sports together?*

It is now generally accepted that boys and girls in the prepubertal years can play sports together without increased risk of physical injury. Because puberty gives boys an advantage in both strength and size, safety and fairness then dictate that boys and girls should no longer compete against each other. However, if there is no team for girls in a certain sport, a girl should be allowed to compete for a position on an all-boys team. It is still controversial whether the reverse should also be allowed, however.

6. *Are injuries more likely to occur in certain sports than in others?*

Football is implicated in more serious injuries than any other sport. In addition, there are relatively high injury rates in wrestling, gymnastics, and ice hockey.[7] Only about 5% of sports injuries involve fractures. By far the greatest number of injuries–two thirds of the total–are sprains and strains. Knee injuries are the most common serious injury in major sports. Boxing carries such a high risk of brain damage that no young person should participate in that sport.

In collision sports, the risk of significant injury can be minimized when the programs are properly supervised. Participation in a relatively high-risk sport stops short of recklessness when there is good coaching and equipment and the rules are adjusted to protect the young athlete. When children need intense physical activity, supervised activities may be preferable to reckless pursuits divorced from sports and any type of supervision.

7. *Are sports activities too stressful for young children?*

Sports activities involve children in stressful situations. However, this is part of learning and development. Competition is a part of all phases of everyday living, including sports. Unreasonable pressure to win creates an unhealthy stress and distorts a child's developing value system, but total avoidance of stress undermines learning and growth.

One study of stress responses demonstrated that the stress of performing a music solo was far greater than that created by participants in a sports contest. Stress can be managed in sports through a number of simple steps. Children should be placed in groups that maintain a narrow range of age levels and degrees of skill. When possible, only players of similar height, weight, ability, and maturity should be matched as opponents in contact sports. The rules of a sport can be changed to make it fairer for all to play.

The main source of stress in the young athlete is the pressure to win. Sadly, many coaches and parents place winning above the values of play and learning. A child's performance should be measured by the yardstick of effort. He or she will respond better to rewards for trying hard, or for gaining skills, than to punishment and criticism for losing. The solution to this problem is the withdrawal of the adult pressure, not the withdrawal of the child from the sport.

8. *How should I select the right coach for my child?*

The best coach for a child is one who emphasizes having FUN. The development of a child's sports skills should be of secondary importance and winning only an incidental benefit. The coach should be familiar with and ascribe to the tenets put forth in the "Bill of Rights for Young Athletes"[8] (Table 3). He or she should be knowledgeable about the sport being coached and should be motivated to be a good coach, not just coerced to fill in as a leader. Many youth sport coaches participate in coaching certification programs (eg, American Coaching Effectiveness Program or the National Youth Sport Coaches Association program[9,11]).

9. *Can my child be excused from physical education class?*

Most of the young people who request this of their parents are the ones who need the physical activity the most. If medical problems interfere with optimal performance, the child should receive treatment (eg, for exercise-induced asthma), rather than be excluded from physical activity. The child with an acute injury should have a rehabilitation program prescribed and performed during the regularly scheduled class rather than avoid physical education while recovering. Most schools provide adaptive physical education for children with disabilities. With the exception of an acute or contagious illness, it is hard to imagine a valid reason for excusing a child from some form of a physical education program.

10. *How do I know if my child's pain is real?*

A complaint of pain should always be accepted as legitimate. The idea that there is a "legitimate" amount of pain for a given injury should be discarded. Each individual has a different pain threshold. In general, pain threshold varies with age (the younger the child, the lower the pain threshold). Pain serves a warning function for acute injury. The intensity of pain an individual feels is affected by a number of variables including age, gender, culture, fear, and anxiety.

The decision as to whether children should continue an activity if they are experiencing pain is more difficult. Before age 6 or 7, a child is not capable of understanding that pain may be acceptable in achieving an outcome benefit (ie, the pain of an immunization injection is worth the long-term protection). All complaints of pain before middle childhood should prompt discontinuance of the activity that produces the pain. After that age, if an athlete clearly wants to return to an activity and there is absolutely no functional disability, he or she may be allowed to do so. However, one must be very careful with an athlete that has a high pain threshold. If the pain is persistent, a medical evaluation should be performed.[10]

REFERENCES

1. Murphy P. Youth fitness testing: a matter of health or performance? *Phys Sportsmed.* 1986;14(5):189-190
2. Rarick GL. Concepts of motor learning: implications for skill development in children. In: Albinson JG, Andrew GM, eds. *Child in Sport and Physical Activity.* Baltimore, MD: University Park Press; 1976:203-217
3. Bailey D. The growing child and the need for physical activity. In: Albinson JG, Andrew GM, eds. *Child in Sport and Physical Activity.* Baltimore, MD: University Park Press; 1976:88-91
4. Shepard R. *Physical Activity and Growth.* Chicago, IL: Year Book Medical Publishers; 1982:198-201
5. Weltman A, Janney C, Rians CB. The effects of hydraulic resistance strength training in prepubertal males. *Med Sci Sports Exerc.* 1986;18(6):629-638
6. Rowland TW. Aerobic response to endurance training in prepubescent children: a critical analysis. *Med Sci Sports Exerc.* 1985;17(5):493-497
7. Garrick JG, Requa RK. Injuries in high school sports. *Pediatrics.* 1978;61:465-469
8. Martens R, et al. *Coaching Young Athletes.* Champaign, IL: Human Kinetics Publishers Inc; 1981
9. American Coaching Effectiveness Program, Box 5076, Champaign, IL 61820, (217) 351-5076
10. Schechter NL. Pain: acknowledging it, assessing it, treating it. *Contemp Pediatr.* 1987;4(7):16-46
11. National Youth Sports Coaches Association, 2611 Old Okeechobee Road, West Palm Beach, FL 33409

SUGGESTED READING

American Academy of Pediatrics, Committee on Psychosocial Aspects of Child and Family Health. *Guidelines for Health Supervision.* Elk Grove Village, IL: American Academy of Pediatrics; 1988

Kirshenbaum JS, Sullivan R. Hold on there, America. *Sports Illustrated.* 1983;58(5):60-74

Michener JA. *Sports in America.* New York, NY: Random House; 1976

Where to turn for sports injury statistics. *Phys Sportsmed.* 1987; 15(4):179-181

Table 1. Anticipatory Guidance: Physical Activity and Sports

Age	Recommendations
2 months	Caution parents about the risks of infant swim classes because of water intoxication, seizures, and transmission of gastroenteritis.
4 months	Advise parents that they need not enroll their children in an infant exercise program. There is no evidence that passive or active exercise at this age promotes any physical advantage.
6 months to 12 months	Discuss water safety, especially the importance of always accompanying the infant when near the water. Discuss pool safety, if appropriate. Encourage unstructured free play with age-appropriate toys.
15 months	Advise parents never to leave a child unsupervised in or near a swimming pool, lake, river, or ditch. "Knowing how to swim" does not make a child water safe at this age. Suggest active play: chasing, dancing, splashing in water, throwing and kicking a ball, and other supervised physical activities. Parents should provide freedom to explore in safety. Encourage parents to limit television viewing. (See AAP brochure on Television and the Family)
18 months	Reinforce water safety. Promote play, both quiet and active (eg, chase and hide). Reinforce limited television viewing.

Table 1. Anticipatory Guidance: Physical Activity and Sports
(continued)

Age	Recommendations
24 months	Reinforce water safety. Provide space and encouragement for physical activities such as climbing, running, and outdoor exploration. Reinforce limited television viewing.
3 years	Encourage active play. Discourage passive activities such as watching TV. Play groups may provide good opportunities to learn and gain experience. Reinforce water safety.
4 years	A child may participate in swimming instruction classes. While in or near the water, the child should always be watched without interruption by a responsible adult who can swim. Supervise the child when riding a bike or playing near the street. Enforce the use of helmets and protective pads. Take exploratory walks and outings to new places.
5 years	Do not allow the child to ride a tricycle or bicycle with training wheels in the street; enforce the use of a helmet and protective pads. Watch the child without interruption while in or near the water; teach child to swim. Introduce concepts of fitness and endurance and their possible relationship to subsequent cardiovascular disease. Limit television viewing time.
6 years	Children should maintain appropriate weight and engage regularly in physical activity. Parents should spend active time with their children, on a daily basis if possible. Consider community youth sports and family physical activities such as biking, running, and swimming. If child is involved in organized sports, ensure that the coach emphasizes learning and fun play rather than winning. Caution against trampoline use. Reinforce bicycle safety, including use of helmets and pads.

Table 1. Anticipatory Guidance: Physical Activity and Sports *(continued)*

Age	Recommendations
8 years	Engage regularly in physical activity. Limit passive activities such as TV viewing and video games. Maintain appropriate weight. Practice bicycle, skating, and skateboard safety, including use of helmets and protective padding. Strength training is appropriate with proper supervision, particularly for the committed athlete. Endurance training is of some limited benefit. Avoid use of trampolines.
10 years	Maintain appropriate weight. Engage in regular physical activity. Limit television viewing and video games. Avoid use of trampolines. Practice bicycle and skateboard safety, including the necessity of wearing helmets and pads.
12 years	Maintain appropriate weight. Engage regularly in physical activities, such as walking, running, swimming, tennis, and bike riding. Advise on sports conditioning, fluids, weight training, and weight gain or loss. Check on physical activity opportunities for handicapped adolescents. Wear a helmet for any riding activities.
14 years	Maintain appropriate weight. Engage in regular physical activity. Discuss benefits of physical fitness. Avoid illicit ergogenic and stimulant drugs with special emphasis on anabolic steroids. For athletes, discuss conditioning and protective equipment.
16 years	Reinforce maintenance of appropriate weight, regular physical activity, and benefits of fitness. If appropriate, reinforce athletic conditioning and avoidance of drugs.
18 years	Reinforce maintenance of appropriate weight, regular physical activity, and benefits of fitness. If appropriate, reinforce athletic conditioning and avoidance of drugs.

Table 1. Anticipatory Guidance: Physical Activity and Sports
(continued)

Age	Recommendations
20 years	Reinforce maintenance of appropriate weight, regular physical activity, and benefits of fitness. If appropriate, reinforce athletic conditioning and avoidance of drugs.

Table 2. Aerobic Value of Selected Sports*

Individual Sports		Team Sports	
Cycling (long and middle distances)	+ + +	Baseball	+
Gymnastics	+	Basketball	+ +
Horseback Riding	−	Soccer	+ +
Running		Football	+ +
sprint	+	Ice Hockey	+ +
middle distance	+ + +	Volleyball	+
long distance	+ + +		
Skiing			
downhill	+ +		
x-country	+ + +		
Swimming	+ + +		
Tennis	+ +		
Walking	+ +		
Weight-lifting	−		
Wrestling/Judo	+ +		

+ and − = Relative Aerobic Value
*Extracted from Bar-Or. *Pediatric Sports Medicine for the Practitioner.* New York, NY: Springer-Verlag; 1983

Table 3. Bill of Rights for Young Athletes*

Right to participate in sports.

Right to participate at a level commensurate with each child's maturity and ability.

Right to have qualified adult leadership.

Right to play as a child and not as an adult.

Right of children to share in the leadership and decision-making of their sport participation.

Right to participate in safe and healthy environments.

Right to proper preparation for participation in sports.

Right to an equal opportunity to strive for success.

Right to be treated with dignity.

Right to have fun in sports.

---

*Reprinted with permission from American Alliance for Health, Physical Education, Recreation, and Dance. *Parents' Complete Guide to Youth Sports.* 1989.

CHAPTER 2

MATURATION

Physical and psychosocial maturation has a direct bearing on what sports activities and exercise are appropriate for children at different ages. In response to the need of parents to feel that they are properly stimulating their child, new commercial ventures are always evolving. Questions are frequently on the minds of parents regarding the appropriateness of different activities for their children. The responsible physician should be prepared to provide guidance for appropriate activities for children and young adults. What follows is designed to provide clinicians with background information with which they can counsel families.

Infants

Skeletal muscle accounts for approximately 25% of weight in a full-term baby. Late in gestation, the number of muscle fibers increases, but most subsequent postnatal growth is due to hypertrophy of muscle cells and fibers, with only small increases in the numbers of cells.

Fatty tissue averages 22% of total body mass in normal newborns. Although the number of fat cells increases in the first year of life, this appears to be independent of diet and activity. Hypertrophy of fat cells apparently is the consequence of excess calorie intake. The adage that fat babies make fat adults cannot be supported by the available evidence.

In infancy, the predominant neuromuscular responses are reflex in nature. As the infant progresses through the first year of life, more and more responses are learned. Although there are certainly inherited individual differences, most of the activity at this age can be attributed to an inherent need to develop self-sufficiency skills (ie, sitting, walking, and feeding). Natural curiosity and the drive towards self-sufficiency motivate the infant in virtually all activities.[1,2] When properly integrated with the opportunity for learning, this inherent drive will help ensure the child's motor and psychosocial development.

Although it is true that deprivation will impede the progress of the young child, it does not necessarily follow that increased stimulation will develop advanced skills. There is evidence that conditioned responses can be elicited in the newborn period.[1] However, there are virtually no data suggesting that this has any long-term benefit for sports skills or exercise efficiency.

Toddlers and Preschoolers

Toddlers and preschool children are still highly motivated by their intrinsic arousal-seeking drive.[1] They are usually seeking self-sufficiency skills such as walking, talking, and self-feeding. The child is naturally motivated to learn through active free play while experimenting in different techniques to learn skills. Until the age of 3, most of these learning processes are self-centered; children have little capacity to adopt socialization skills necessary to interact with their peers. Between 3 and 5 years of age, self-directed skills such as visuospatial perception, motor manipulation, body positioning, and ability to release thrown objects improve markedly. What little data have been developed have shown operant learning (response to reinforcement techniques for learning) for sports skills to be of minimal benefit. Toddlers who have practiced ball throwing show virtually no greater skills than non-ball-throwing toddlers when they reach school age. Adult interventions to teach specific skills to children of this age tend to stifle the self-seeking ability of children in play to develop their own proficiency levels.

Understanding that there are individual variations in maturity, one can say that by approximately 3 years of age, children are able to take on the more complex learning tasks in play with other preschoolers. These children appear to learn best when provided a safe, unstructured play environment. At this age, children benefit from the socialization process but are poorly equipped to handle the more complex skills required for team play.

It is not until approximately age 5 years that children begin to develop the cognitive thinking skills necessary for complex sports activities and safety. They still function at a very concrete level. That is, it is not uncommon for children who have enjoyed parent/tot swimming classes later to develop fear of the water because it is the first time that they have recognized the consequences of being under water.

Skeletal muscle as a percentage of body composition remains relatively constant, whereas the percentage of body fat tends to decrease in the preschool child. Children of this age rarely exercise themselves to the point of maximum oxygen uptake (VO_2max) or power output. This may be because of the lower biomechanical and metabolic efficiency in children, compared to adults, which is necessary to maximally exert oneself. However, normal play activity stimulates the aerobic capacities adequately so that by the time children enter school, their VO_2max relative to their body size is nearly the same as later in life.

The cardiorespiratory system is small for the body size of the prepubertal child relative to that of the pubertal child or adult. Prepubertal children appear to compensate for this by the development of a greater amount of tachypnea and tachycardia in response to exercise than do older children and adults.

School-Aged Children

The ability of the 5- to 6-year-old child to learn motor skills increases rapidly. For instance, farsightedness caused by the spheroidal shape of the eyeball, and difficulty tracking fast moving objects are resolving by age 6 or 7. Evidence now indicates that mature patterns of throwing behavior can be attained by the time a child is 6 or 7 years old.

Children have difficulty integrating information from different sources. Consequently, there are frequently problems with laterality, directionality, and body image. Certain sports with complex movement patterns require a good deal of coordination, strength, and power. Many children before ages 7 or 8 do not have the skills necessary to learn these complex movements, which may result in poor performance or failure. By waiting until a child is 9 or 10, the added maturity may result in more rapid learning and success in the activity. A good example of a sports adaptation to these limitations is the introduction of "T" ball in community programs, in which children hit a baseball perched on a stand so that they will not have to deal with direction and velocity of a pitched ball in the process of learning to bat.

In the middle childhood years, reflex times are constantly decreasing and balance skills are improving. Sports involving a heavy emphasis on these skills (ie, basketball or football) may be more successfully introduced to the 9- or 10-year-old child.

The attention span of children of this age is sufficiently short that they learn most efficiently in small groups with short, frequent instruction periods. Their ability to concentrate in large groups for extended, infrequent practices is minimal, often resulting in frustration and loss of interest. The optimum age for instruction remains controversial and is best judged by the specific skills to be taught and by the individual maturity of the child. The child's ability to function in the classroom, socialize with peers, and perform motor tasks at home may be appropriate indicators.

The maximum aerobic power of the active child at this age relative to body size is surprisingly high. Children who are involved in regular unstructured play often maintain a VO$_2$max/kg as high or higher than most adults.[3]

Before puberty, increased aerobic training beyond usual play may enhance maximal aerobic power. However, the advantage to the prepubertal child of extended periods of exercise to improve conditioning is minimal and is won only at the cost of intense effort needed to bring about these improvements.

The muscular system is adaptable to training effects. Properly conducted strength training has been shown to improve strength in the prepubertal child. Because balance and other proprioceptive skills are still evolving, careful supervision is a must for any strength-training program. These children may be more at risk for injury from free weights than fixed weights such as Universal gyms and Nautilus-type equipment.

The skeletal system is still immature. Growing cartilage in epiphyseal plates is vulnerable to repeated stress and trauma in the prepubertal and early pubertal child. The long-term consequences of overuse trauma (see Chapter 12) on growth and later disability are not known. However, anatomic changes in such epiphyseal areas have been demonstrated in children with overuse syndromes. One of the more striking examples involved Little League pitchers who demonstrated epicondylitis of the humerus. The frequency of this injury resulted in rule changes limiting the amount and type of pitches these youngsters may throw in a game, and the condition is rarely seen now. Long bones are not completely ossified and may be more vulnerable to minor trauma resulting in fractures and overuse syndromes.[4] Ten percent to 15% of such injuries involve the epiphyseal plate, and 20% of those may result in growth disturbances of the bone. In spite of these frailties, prepubertal children in collision sports are less likely to suffer serious injury than postpubertal children. This probably relates to the fact that the force of the collision (when children weigh less and are not traveling fast) is not as great at the earlier age. A serious injury is less likely to result from a collision between two 70-lb children than between two 250-lb adolescents.

Adolescents

The zenith of learning sports skills develops in the early stages of adolescence and continues throughout adolescence. However, most people recognize the inherent awkwardness and clumsiness of the pubertal child, which may reflect that the body is temporarily poorly equipped to process the newly learned skills.

Maturity assessment is an important part of the preparticipation evaluation for the pubertal child.[5] Maturity rating is most important for participators in collision sports, most of whom are boys. However, some girls do compete in these sports, and they should have maturity assessments performed. In the 11- to 15-year age range, there are great variations in the physical maturity of children. Maturity assessment is most easily done through the evaluation of pubic hair development using the Tanner scales as a guide (Chapter 4, Figs. 2 and 3). Athletes of either sex who are skeletally immature (less than Stage 3, Tanner rating) should be either discouraged from participating in, or at least warned about the increased risks of playing, collision sports when they would be competing against athletes who are physically more mature. The musculoskeletal system appears to be most vulnerable during this period of peak height velocity (Tanner Stage 3). Studies indicate that the incidence of epiphyseal injuries peaks during puberty. The epiphyseal plate is weaker than surrounding tissue at this age, perhaps due to biochemical changes that occur during rapid growth. Overuse syndromes (eg, patellofemoral syndrome and Osgood-Schlatter disease) frequently begin to occur at this time. Normal recreational activity at this age usually causes no problems, but intense prolonged training or involvement in collision sports may increase risk for development of overuse syndromes. Many conscientious coaches decrease the intensity of training during this period of rapid growth (see Chapter 12).

For pubertal children to maintain the degree of VO_2max exhibited by prepubertal children, planned aerobic exercise is necessary. The cardiorespiratory system grows disproportionately larger than the rest of the body, thereby making exercise more economical and efficient. Increased emphasis on strength training and developing muscle endurance also contributes to efficiency during exercise and competition. It is possible to participate in exercise that maintains aerobic fitness without going to the extremes that may risk overuse injury to the musculoskeletal system.

Gender differences of musculoskeletal development affecting competition occur during puberty. Boys acquire proportionately greater musculoskeletal mass than do girls. The boy's shoulder girdle and the girl's pelvis grow disproportionately larger, resulting in mismatched upper and lower body strength. It is not surprising that girls have more difficulty with pull-ups than boys. Aerobic capacity and proprioceptive skills are probably not significant factors as far as safety is concerned. However, what differences do occur may impact on performance inequities. Girls are possibly at greater risk of injury in contact/collision sports with boys. However, boys who mature skeletally more slowly than girls may be at greater risk of injury if competing against physically mature girls who may temporarily have more mature skeletal systems.

Young Adults

As the child progresses through adolescence, there is further refinement in learning and proprioceptive skills. More complex tasks are easier to learn and the ability to discriminate individual items in the environment increases. These athletes are more equipped to look at the details of a sport skill and to concentrate on them to improve overall performance.

There is a continuing need to maintain exercise levels that support muscle strength and endurance, cardiorespiratory endurance, flexibility, and body composition. The continuation of good aerobic fitness may be a component of good cardiovascular health in the future. By late adolescence, the musculoskeletal system begins to reach maturity. Epiphyseal injuries become less frequent. Strength training to maintain musculoskeletal fitness and maximize performance is essential for virtually all sports.

Unfortunately, the sports system in this country favors the elite athlete. Awards and trophies are usually awarded to only the most valuable and most improved athletes. The emphasis on winning, in high schools, overshadows the goal of participation in sports for all children, thereby limiting participation to all but the most gifted athletes. The physician must find individual motivational factors for the adolescent who does not excel in sports to continue regular exercise.

REFERENCES

1. Shepard RJ. Growth of motor skills. Motivating the child toward physical activity. In: Shepard RJ, ed. *Physical Activity and Growth.* Chicago, IL: Year Book Medical Publishers; 1982:107-123,233-245
2. Rarick GL. Concepts of motor learning: implications for skill development in children. In: Albinson JG, Andrew GM, eds. *Child in Sport and Physical Activity.* Baltimore, MD: University Park Press; 1976:203-217
3. Bar-Or O. *Pediatric Sports Medicine for the Practitioner: From Physiologic Principles to Clinical Applications.* New York, NY: Springer-Verlag; 1983
4. Royer P. Growth and development of bony tissue. In: Davis JA, Dobbing J, eds. *Scientific Foundations of Pediatrics.* Philadelphia, PA: WB Saunders Co; 1974:chap 21
5. Caine DJ, Broekhoff J. Maturity assessment: a viable preventive measure against physical and psychological insult to the young athlete? *Phys Sportsmed.* 1987;15(3):67-70,73-75,78-80

CHAPTER 3

THE FEMALE ATHLETE

In the not-too-distant past, girls and women generally were discouraged not only from sports participation but from exercising in general. The myth that it was "unfeminine" and that it would produce "unsightly muscle bulk" prevailed. Opportunities for females were few. In fact, in the 1896 Olympics, female participants were not allowed to compete. As late as 1968, only 14% of the participants were women, and it was not until 1984 that women were allowed to participate in the Olympic marathon.

Today we should actively encourage girls to become involved in exercise and sports. Opportunities for female participation have increased tremendously. Girls can now reap all the same physical and emotional benefits that boys have. It is no longer considered unfeminine to desire to win or to strive for achievement goals in sports. Female athletes have been found to have a more positive body image and demonstrate higher psychologic well-being than their sedentary counterparts.[1]

Body Composition

The body's composition usually is divided into lean body mass and nonessential fat. Lean body mass is the fat-free tissue together with some essential (structural) lipids. The differences in body composition, physiologic values, and actual performance between males and females are small until adolescence.[2]

After puberty, the percentage of body fat in females is usually greater than in males. Since there has been no systematic evaluation of the body fat content of representative samples from the general population, there are no precise norms or standards for comparison purposes.

Whether individuals gravitate towards sports with which their body composition is most compatible or whether the sport tailors the athlete's body composition is not known.

Aerobic Function and Performance

The physiologic responses of males and females to endurance stress are similar.[3-5] In addition, there do not appear to be differences in muscle fiber type and ability to metabolize fat.[2] Of note is that most physiologic variables, when expressed in absolute terms (ie, VO_2max in liters per minute), are lower in women, but when expressed relative to body size and composition (ie, VO_2max in mL/kg fat-free weight/min), the differences are slight.[2]

Muscle Strength and Strength Training

The glycolytic oxidative enzymes of male and female muscle possess the same adaptability to training,[6,7] and we see the same physiologic ability of male and female muscle to adapt to strength training (also known as "resistance training" and "weight training").[8] Why, then, the apparent discrepancy between male and female muscle strength and bulk?

Wilmore[9] states that the average upper body strength of the female is 30% to 50% that of males, whereas the lower body strength of the female is 70% of males. Yet, strength levels of women are found to be similar to or even greater (legs and hips) than that of men when strength is related to lean mass weight rather than total body weight.[10,11] Since the increase in strength of the upper and lower body for both sexes is similar with proper training,[12] the theory that androgens in males principally account for their increased strength has been questioned.[2,12-14] Many of the differences noted in the past may have had to do with social and cultural changes that occurred after puberty: females were expected to do less upper body work, and hence, did not continue to develop muscle strength after puberty. Corrected to lean body mass, women may be of equivalent strength, but this cannot be done on the playing field; hence, the male's usual advantage.

With a sufficient increase in muscle work, a male's muscles increase in bulk after puberty. This is felt to be secondary to circulating testosterone levels.[3,10,16] Women have much lower levels of testosterone and, hence, can increase strength without concomitant increases in bulk.[3,12,15,17,18] Muscle bulk is not correlated with strength.[3,16]

Fears still abound regarding strength training in females–unsightly muscularity ("bulk"), reduced motor coordination, decreased flexibility, and speed. Many females also fear the label "unfeminine" and believe training is inappropriate behavior, resulting in an inappropriate goal–strength. Still others believe that females are not capable of tolerating or adapting to the rigors of intensive training. These fears and beliefs have not been sustained by scientific scrutiny.

The benefits of strength training include increased strength (of bones, ligaments, and musculotendinous units), power, and muscle endurance. This form of training is the major reason for the increased performance of athletes today. Strength training is one of the most neglected areas of the female American athlete's development.[19,20] For most female athletes today, strength training is only an optional part of their total conditioning, although it is necessary for all athletes–males and females–to achieve their maximal performance.

In the past, it was often assumed that females were at increased risk of injury because of less strength than their male counterparts. There is no clear relationship between strength, performance, and injury risks.[21] Hence, although separate competitions for postpubertal males and females may be fairer, they may be no more safe than coeducational participation.[21]

Gynecologic Considerations

Female athletes may have many gynecologic concerns, eg, delay of menarche, menstrual irregularities, amenorrhea, infertility, contraception, premenstrual syndrome, menstrual cramps, and breast-related complaints. Some athletes may feel that they are immune to normal medical problems and may conclude (especially with menstrual difficulties) that these are due to their physical activity level. This can be a dangerous assumption and evaluation should be encouraged.

Menstrual Physiology

The menstrual cycle involves a complex interaction between a woman's hypothalamus, pituitary gland, ovaries, and uterus. The hypothalamus produces and secretes gonadotropin-releasing hormone (GnRH), which subsequently stimulates the pituitary gland to produce and secrete two gonadotropins, follicle-stimulating hormone (FSH), and luteinizing hormone (LH). The FSH promotes growth of the ovarian follicle and production of estrogen. The LH triggers ovulation, which results in the development of the corpus luteum and production of progesterone.

Estrogen is the initial stimulant for the growth of the endometrium; progesterone subsequently helps to convert the endometrium into a stable mature structure. If no pregnancy ensues, the endometrium is shed about 14 days after ovulation when estrogen and progesterone levels drop.

Menses

Some females feel that menstruation has an adverse effect on their performance,[22] but Fox and Mathews summarized the literature[23] and found that most female athletes exhibit no change in performance during menses. There is no need to change practice or competition schedules.[24] Some evidence suggests that vigorous exercise yields the beneficial effects of less menstrual flow and a subjectively better feeling.[13]

Delayed Menarche

Athletes tend to experience menarche at a later age than do nonathletes.[25-27] Frisch et al[28] stated that athletes who train intensively before menarche begin their menses an average of 2.3 years later than nonathletes, and each year of premenarchal training delays menarche by 0.4 years. Although menarche may be delayed, the appearance of secondary sexual characteristics is not.

Controversy continues as to whether this menarchal delay is self-selected. Some authors suggest that delayed puberty promotes athletic success in certain sports[29]; others suggest that exercise delays puberty.[28] Its etiology most likely is an interaction among several factors, including decreased body fat, physical stress, emotional stress, and nutritional factors (including anorexia and bulimia).

Evaluation should be encouraged if by age 14 the female has no signs of secondary sexual development (breast, axillary hair, pubic hair) or if by age 16 there are no menses.[30] Work-up for delayed menarche or puberty should include a pelvic examination; tests for serum FSH, LH, thyroid-stimulating hormone (TSH), and prolactin; roentgenographic bone age (if pubertal development is delayed, interrupted, or incomplete); and chromosome analysis if Turner syndrome or other chromosomal anomaly is suspected.

In order to rule out outflow tract abnormalities, a trial with 10 mg per day of oral medroxyprogesterone acetate for 7 days should be instituted. Withdrawal bleeding generally occurs within 3 or 4 days of completion of this regimen, and this serves to confirm that the genital tract is intact. If no withdrawal bleeding occurs, referral to a gynecologist would be wise.

Girls less than 16 years should be encouraged to be active regardless of menarchal delay, as there is no evidence of any significant health risk. Once 16, replacement estrogen should be considered to prevent osteoporosis.

Menstrual Dysfunction

It is believed that menstrual dysfunction is more common in athletes,[30] but studies of amenorrheic athletes are fraught with lack of standard definitions, poor subject selection, inadequate body composition measurements, and little consideration for preexisting menstrual irregularities.[31] Menstrual dysfunction in athletes is felt to include a spectrum of changes in the menstrual cycle that may be a continuum of interruptions of the hypothalamic–pituitary ovarian–axis.

"Primary amenorrhea" means that a female has never had a menstrual period. "Secondary amenorrhea" indicates that a female has menstruated, but has had no more than two menses in the last 12 months. "Oligomenorrhea"[24] denotes fewer than six menses in a consecutive 12-month period. All females who skip menstruating for 2 or more months and all who menstruate irregularly (more often than every 25 days or less often than every 35 days counting from the first day of one period to the first day of the next) should be examined, regardless of whether they exercise.[32] To assume that menstrual difficulties are secondary to exercise is dangerous and creates an unnecessary delay in evaluation.

The exact etiology of the disruption of this complex menstrual cycle in athletes is not known, but it is probably multifactoral. Nutritional alterations, weight loss, decreased body fat, physical stress, emotional stress, and transient and/or chronic alterations in hormone levels all may play a role.

Eumenorrheic Athletes

Overtrained athletes have been shown to have blunted responses to insulin-induced hypoglycemia.[33] This represents hypothalamic dysfunction. Female athletes have been found to have a reduction in their frequency and amplitude of LH pulsation[34]; this may be the first clue to early menstrual dysfunction in a normally menstruating athlete.[32] In addition, eumenorrheic athletes can experience either a shortened luteal phase or anovulation.[35] Shortening of the luteal phase is most subtle but does result in decreases in production of progesterone.[36] Infertility is the only abnormality reported to be associated with this condition.[32]

Athletes With Irregular Menses

Anovulation is likely to result in irregular menstrual periods or oligomenorrhea. When anovulation exists the ovaries can continue to produce estrogen but no progesterone is produced. Hence, unopposed estrogen stimulates the endometrium and breasts, which can result in more serious concerns—endometrial hyperplasia and possibly increased risk of breast cancer.[37]

Amenorrheic Athletes

Anovulatory women who become hypoestrogenic are often amenorrheic. The lack of estrogen produced by the ovaries is probably a result of inadequate gonadotropin stimulation. Secondary dangers include osteoporosis and atrophic vaginitis. Few of these athletes will present with symptoms that are usually associated with estrogen deficiency—

hot flashes, emotional lability, and dyspareunia (secondary to vaginal dryness)–but will present with absence of menses.

Evaluation of Menstrual Dysfunction

A history, a physical examination, and a laboratory evaluation are required to rule out pregnancy (the most common cause of amenorrhea), prolactin-secreting tumor, premature menopause (ovarian failure), and an endocrine disorder. The breasts should be checked for galactorrhea. Initial blood tests should include (if a pregnancy test is negative), prolactin, TSH, T_3 resin uptake, FSH, and LH. An elevated prolactin level requires further investigation for a possible prolactin-secreting tumor of the pituitary gland.

Elevated FSH and LH indicate ovarian failure, and, if the female is less than 30 years old, a blood karyotype should be obtained because of the possibility of Turner syndrome.

Elevated LH and FSH (or the LH/FSH ratio) in a patient who is hirsute and has oligomenorrhea means that circulating androgens should be measured. If these are elevated, polycystic ovarian syndrome is likely.

If LH and FSH levels are less than 10 IU/mL even with normal prolactin, radiologic evaluation of the pituitary gland should be pursued,[38] since all pituitary tumors do not secrete prolactin.

After initial studies are drawn and pregnancy is ruled out, a progesterone challenge test could be instituted. A prescription for oral medroxyprogesterone acetate should be given (10 mg per day for 5 days), and, if estrogen has been present, the athlete will have withdrawal bleeding within a few days of completing the progesterone. If no withdrawal occurs, the female has low levels of circulating estrogens and may require replacement therapy.

Treatment

Data on the reversibility of exercise-associated menstrual dysfunction are unavailable, although many physicians believe menstrual irregularities can be reversed by changes in lifestyle (decreased activity and increased caloric intake). The clinical significance of menstrual dysfunction remains obscure,[30] and the management may be dependent on whether the female athlete desires pregnancy[30] and whether she wishes to decrease her activity level.

Females With Menstrual Irregularities and Positive Progesterone Challenge Test (presence of circulating estrogens)

Since these females have unopposed estrogen, medroxyprogesterone acetate should be given in 5- to 10-mg doses once daily for 10 days at the end of each calendar month. If these females desire contraceptives, birth control pills may be used throughout the whole cycle, as normally prescribed.

Females With Menstrual Irregularities and Negative Progesterone Challenge Test

These females are hypoestrogenic. To protect their bones and vaginal mucosa, they require conjugated estrogens 0.625 mg once daily for the first 25 days and medroxyprogesterone acetate (5 mg) once daily on days 14 to 25 each calendar month. Low-dosage birth control pills can be substituted for convenience or if pregnancy is not desired.

Osteoporosis and Amenorrheic Athletes

Osteoporosis is a relative deficiency of the mineral content of bone. Studies indicate a decrease in the bone density of amenorrheic athletes.[39-41] This effect is felt to be secondary to decreased circulating estrogen.[39,40] Whether these young women are at increased risk of fractures has not yet been determined, but there is at least a theoretical risk. Spine densities in the lower spine are primarily affected, at least compared to bone densities seen in the forearm.[41]

Risk factors for osteoporosis include decreased estrogen levels (as noted above), sedentary life style, Caucasian race, positive family history of osteoporosis, low weight-for-height ratio, poor diet (low calcium, high caffeine, high alcohol, high protein, and high phosphate), and cigarette smoking.

Peak bone mass is attained in both men and women at about age 35.[42] To maximize peak bone mass, we should encourage good nutritional health in youngsters. We should encourage active life styles early on, and give replacement estrogen to hypoestrogenic women. Nilssen et al[43] stated that physical activity that begins before growth ends seems to result in higher-than-average bone mineral content and increased dimensions of the bones of the lower limbs.

If an adult female has a 2-year history of amenorrhea, it is suggested that the bone mineral content of her vertebrae be estimated.[42] Either dual-beam photon absorptiometry or computerized axial tomography can be used for measurement.

Other menstrual disorders—heavy bleeding, clotting, and spotting—are usually symptoms of other conditions (unrelated to exercise) and also should be investigated.[24]

Infertility

The rate of infertility in athletes is said to be the same as in nonathletes.[44] Females with menstrual dysfunction—luteal phase insufficiency, menstrual irregularity (with probable anovulation), and/or amenorrhea—probably will have difficulty conceiving. Should they wish to become pregnant and still are infertile after a year of unprotected intercourse, they should consult a gynecologist experienced in infertility problems.[30]

Contraceptives

If interested in contraceptives, the alternatives for the athlete are the same as for the nonathlete and should be decided on by medical history, fertility plans, and frequency of intercourse.[30]

Birth control pills can increase blood volume and cardiac output, but their effect on exercise performance is not known.[24] At the present time, there is no obvious reason to use or prohibit use of the pill in exercising females.

Females who exercise and who have decreased body fat usually have favorable plasma lipid and lipoprotein concentrations while taking oral contraceptives. These exercise-associated changes partially compensate for adverse changes caused by birth control pills.

The diaphragm, if properly fitted, should not interfere with exercise.

The intrauterine device is not advised in very young women who plan to have children because of the increased risk of pelvic infection. Increased cramping, abdominal pain, and bleeding are seen,[24] and these problems have the potential for interfering with physical performance.

Premenstrual Syndrome (PMS)

Premenstrual syndrome is a commonly encountered problem for women for several days before onset of their menses. This syndrome has various symptoms including anxiety, depression, fluid retention, and hunger. The etiology is not known. There is no evidence that PMS worsens with exercise,[24] and there is no contraindication to participation with this syndrome. Treatment with spironolactone beginning 3 to 4 days before anticipation of symptoms may help to prevent or relieve the symptoms.

Dysmenorrhea

Menstrual cramps are a great concern to athletes because they can be disabling. Yet, there is no reason to avoid exercise during early menses when dysmenorrhea occurs. Exercise may be beneficial because of distraction, exercise-induced production of pain-killing endorphins, and production of vasodilating prostaglandins.[30] Dysmenorrhea should be aggressively treated with a prostaglandin inhibitor such as ibuprofen.

Breasts

Although the breasts are in a seemingly unprotected location, few athletic injuries have been reported.[24] Minor concerns include nipple abrasions (seen in males also) and breast or shoulder pain, which may be secondary to insufficient support of pendulous breast tissue.

Nipple abrasions result from loss of the epithelial covering of the nipple usually from rubbing of an overlying shirt. Band-aids over the nipples can be preventive and protective.

Shoulder and breast pain can be prevented by use of a supportive brassiere. Small-breasted women may opt to go without breast support without adverse consequences.

The breasts are made up of mostly fat tissue, hence exercises neither increase tone nor size. The pectoralis muscles which underlie the breasts can be strengthened and give an illusion of increased breast size. If body fat percentage is decreased, breast size may decrease.

REFERENCES

1. Chalip L, Villiger J, Duignan P. Sex role identity in a select sample of women field hockey players. *Int J Sport Psychol.* 1980; 11:240-248
2. Berg K. Aerobic function in female athletes. *Clin Sports Medicine.* 1984;3:779-789
3. Drinkwater BL. Physiological response of women to exercise. *Exer Sports Review.* 1973;1:125-153
4. Plowman S. Physiological characteristics of female athletes. *Res Q Am Assoc Health Phys Educ.* 1974;45:349-362
5. Wilmore JH, Brown CH. Physiologic profiles of women distance runners. *Med Sci Sports.* 1974;6:178-181
6. Costill DL, Evans W, Daniels J, Fink W, Krahenbuhl G. Skeletal muscle enzymes and fiber composition in male and female track athletes. *J Appl Physiol.* 1976;40:149-154

7. Nygaard E, Neilsen E. Skeletal muscle fiber capillarization with extreme endurance training in man. In: Eriksson B, Furberg B, eds. *Swimming Medicine IV.* Baltimore, MD: University Park Press; 1978:282-293

8. Baechle TR: Women in resistance training. *Clin Sports Medicine.* 1984;3:791-808

9. Wilmore JH. The application of science to sport: physiologic profiles of male and female athletes. *Can J Appl Sports Sci.* 1979;4:103-115

10. Berger RA. *Applied Exer Phys.* Philadelphia, PA: Lea and Febiger; 1982

11. Brown CH, Wilmore JH. The effects of maximal resistance training on the strength and body composition of women athletes. *Med Sci Sports.* 1974;6(3):174-177

12. Wilmore JH. Alterations in strength, body composition and anthropometric measurements consequent to a 10-week training program. *Med Sci Sports.* 1974;6:133-138

13. Anderson JL. Women's sports and fitness programs at the US Military Academy. *Phys Sportsmed.* 1979;7:72-80

14. Montoye HJ, Lamphiear DE. Grip and arm strength in males and females age 10 to 69. *Res Q Am Assoc Health Phys Educ.* 1977;48:109-120

15. Mayhew JL, Gross PM. Body composition changes in young women with high resistance weight training. *Res Q.* 1974; 45(4):433-440

16. Assmussen E. Growth in muscular strength and power. In: Rarick GL, ed. *Physical Activity, Human Growth and Development.* New York, NY: Academic Press; 1973:60-79

17. Morehouse LE, Miller AT. *Physiology of Exercise.* 7th ed. St. Louis, MO: CV Mosby Company; 1976

18. Moulds B, Carter DR, Coleman J, Stone MH. Physical responses of a women's basketball team to a preseason conditioning program. In: Terauds J, ed. *Science in Sports.* Del Mar, CA: Academic Publishers; 1979:203-210

19. O'Shea JP. *Scientific Principles and Methods of Strength Fitness.* 2nd ed. Reading, MA: Addison-Wesley Publishing Company; 1976

20. O'Shea JP, Wegner J. Power weight training and the female athlete. *Phys Sportsmed.* 1981;9(6):109-115,119-120

21. Micheli LJ. *Pediatric and Adolescent Sports Medicine.* Boston, MA: Little, Brown and Company; 1984

22. Bale P, Nelson G. The effects of menstruation on performance of swimmers. *Aust J Sci Med Sport.* 1985;17:19-22

23. Fox EL, Mathews DK. *The Physiological Basis of Physical Education and Athletics.* 3rd ed. Philadelphia, PA: Saunders College Publishing; 1981

24. Hale RW. Factors important to women engaged in vigorous physical activity. In: Strauss RH, ed. *Sports Med.* Philadelphia, PA: Saunders Co; 1984:250-269

25. Malina RM, Harper AB, Avent HH, Campbell DE. Age at menarche in athletes and non-athletes. *Med Sci Sports.* 1973; 5:11-13

26. Malina RM, Spirduso WW, Tate C, Baylor AM. Age at menarche and selected menstrual characteristics in athletes at different competitive levels and in different sports. *Med Sci Sports.* 1978; 10:218-222

27. Warren MP. The effects of exercise on pubertal progression and reproductive function in girls. *J Clin Endocrinol Metab.* 1980; 51:1150-1157

28. Frisch RE, Gotz-Welbergen AV, McArthur JW, et al. Delayed menarche and amenorrhea of college athletes in relation to age of onset of training. *JAMA.* 1981;246:1559-1563

29. Shangold M, Kelly M, Berkely A. The relationship between menarcheal age and adult height. Presented at the Society for Gynecological Investigation, Thirteenth Annual Meeting, Scientific Program and Abstracts; 1983; Abstract

30. Shangold M. Gynecological concerns in the woman athlete. *Clin Sports Medicine.* 1984;3:869-879

31. Loucks AB, Horvath SM. Athletic amenorrhea: a review. *Med Sci Sports.* 1985;17:56-72

32. Shangold MM. How I manage exercise-related menstrual disturbances. *Phys Sportsmed.* 1986;14:113,116,119-120

33. Barron JL, Noakes TD, Levy W, Smith C, Millar RP. Hypothalamic dysfunction in overtrained athletes. *J Clin Endocrinol Metab.* 1985; 60:803-806

34. Cummings DC, Vickovic MM, Wall SR, Fluker MR. Defects in pulsatile LH release in normally menstruating runners. *J Clin Endocrinol Metab.* 1985;60:810-812

35. Prior JC, Cameron K, Yuen BH, Thomas J. Menstrual cycle changes with marathon training: anovulation and short luteal phase. *Can J Appl Sports Sci.* 1982;7:173-177

36. Shangold M, Freeman R, Thysen B, Gatz M. The relationship between long-distance running, plasma progesterone, and luteal phase length. *Fertil Steril.* 1979;31:130-133

37. Gonzalez ER. Chronic anovulation may increase postmenopausal breast cancer risk. *JAMA.* 1983;249:445-446

38. Kustin J, Rebar RW. Addressing concerns of amenorrheic athletes. *The Active Woman, Contemporary Ob-Gyn.* Aug 1986:35-43

39. Cann CE, Martin MC, Genant HK, Jaffe RB. Decreased spinal mineral content in amenorrheic women. *JAMA.* 1984;251:626-629

40. Drinkwater BL, Nilson K, Chesnut CH, Bremner WJ, Shainholtz S, Southworth MB. Bone mineral content of amenorrheic and eumenorrheic athletes. *N Engl J Med.* 1984;311:277-281
41. Marcus R, Cann C, Madvig P, et al. Menstrual function and bone mass in elite women distance runners: endocrine and metabolic features. *Ann Intern Med.* 1985;102:158-163
42. Smith EL, Zook, Sally K. Exercise can reduce bone loss. *The Active Woman, Contemporary Ob-Gyn.* Aug 1986:53-61
43. Nilsson BE, Anderson SM, Havdrup TU, et al. Bone mineral content in ballet dancers and weight lifters. In: Mazess RB, ed. *Proceedings of the Fourth International Conference on Bone Measurement.* Washington, DC: 1980;81-86. National Institutes of Health publication 80-ES1938
44. Shangold MM, Levine HS. The effect of marathon training upon menstrual function. *Am J Obstet Gynecol.* 1982;143:862-869

CHAPTER 4

SPORTS PREPARTICIPATION EXAMINATION

More than 25 million children in the United States participate in organized athletic activities, and there are countless others in physical education classes at school. Although an individualized annual health maintenance physical examination in a physician's office for all these children is ideal, only too often a "locker room" type of mass examination is given to young athletes by a volunteer physician before a competitive season.

Both kinds of "sports physicals," the health maintenance examination in a physician's office and the mass examination, are notoriously ineffective as usually performed in detecting abnormalities that would either affect the athlete's performance or pose an undue risk during athletic participation. If the examination takes place in the physician's office, however, there is an opportunity to offer anticipatory guidance and assess the need for more formal counseling completely unrelated to athletics.[1] About 80% of high school athletes undergoing a sports preparticipation examination have no other annual health assessment by a physician during the school year, so physicians should try to convert the office "sports physical" into a health maintenance examination whenever possible.[2]

A third kind of preparticipation examination—that done by a group of physicians and other personnel in "stations"—has been shown to be very effective in finding physical abnormalities. An advantage of this kind of examination is that it has volunteer physicians who frequently self-select for this task because of an interest in sports medicine and, therefore, a greater knowledge about performing the musculoskeletal component of the examination. A disadvantage is that the physician is not able to administer anticipatory guidance or perform the other components of a health maintenance examination.

The musculoskeletal component of the examination is the most productive part in revealing abnormalities, usually residua of previous injuries, which could lead to other injuries unless rehabilitative exercises are performed. One large study of high school football players indicated that musculoskeletal abnormalities were detected in 10% of them when the examination included a component quite similar to the "two-minute orthopedic examination"[3] (Table 4).

Frequency

The American Academy of Pediatrics has recommended that health maintenance examinations be done at least every two years throughout adolescence, but many schools require an annual sports examination. This is probably because they believe that such a requirement gives them a legal advantage in case of a lawsuit concerning an athletic injury; or they may truly believe that good medical practice requires an annual examination. Certainly, many pediatricians, especially adolescent medicine specialists, believe that health maintenance examinations should be performed annually throughout adolescence.

Laboratory Examinations

Although a urinalysis and hemoglobin/hematocrit have been traditional components of sports examinations, they are not necessary. The urinalysis in particular can produce undue anxiety for adolescents when a 1+ albuminuria is detected, requiring a repeat urinalysis at a later date and usually at least a temporary medical restraint on participation. In one study of preparticipation examinations in which an abnormal urinary protein was detected in 40 of 701 children, further tests revealed that *none* of these children had significant renal or bladder abnormalities. We therefore *do not recommend* a urinalysis as a component of the preparticipation examination, although it may be indicated as part of a health maintenance evaluation.

Although iron-deficiency anemia is not uncommon, it has to be quite severe before the body's compensatory mechanisms fail to maintain an appropriate supply of oxygen to the tissues. There is conflicting evidence about whether mild iron deficiency (ie, hypoferremia without frank anemia) can affect athletic performance. Tests of serum iron or ferritin are expensive and are usually done only on highly competitive national-class female athletes or male marathon runners, two groups of athletes with demonstrated high incidences of iron depletion.[4] Routine hemoglobin/hematocrit determinations are, therefore, *not recommended* for the purposes of a preparticipation evaluation, although they may well be indicated if the examination is also a health maintenance evaluation.

The Medical History

Figure 1 consists of the history component of a sports physical examination form. This is succinct enough to be useful and detailed enough to alert the physician to areas of the physical examination or medical history that need particular attention. Part B of the form is an interim health history that should be obtained in the intervals between complete examinations; this should identify those illnesses and injuries that have occurred since the last examination and may require a physician's evaluation before participation is allowed.

The Examination

The preparticipation health evaluation should be conducted at least 4 to 6 weeks before the beginning of the athletic season so that previous injuries can be identified in time to be treated with rehabilitative exercises in an attempt to prevent reinjury. When the examination is not done on an individual basis in a physician's office, it will frequently be conducted at the school, in which case a "stations" format is most efficient. Regardless of the location of the examination, it should contain *at least* the components outlined below, and the complete musculoskeletal examination (Table 4) should be performed carefully.

Stations Examination

The only requirements are a room large enough to accommodate all the waiting examinees simultaneously and quiet office areas adjacent to the larger room. This arrangement allows all examinees to be given instructions at one time, yet it provides privacy for the portions of the examination requiring the athlete to disrobe.

The area should be divided into examination stations, which should be clearly marked with large printed numbers. Each station should have a chair/desk or a chair and a clipboard. An examination table will be needed at the station where the abdominal examination is done.

Efficient examination of 30 or more athletes within 2 hours requires a team of six: two physicians and four nonphysician medical personnel (nurses, certified athletic trainers, etc.). In addition, the coach of the sport involved should be present to ensure some modicum of order and good attendance.

The athletes must be present, appropriately dressed, at least 10 minutes before the examination is scheduled to begin. Boys should wear gym shorts; girls should wear gym outfits.

The history is the most important aspect of the preparticipation health evaluation. Because medical histories of minors require parental signatures, these forms (Fig. 1) should be completed prior to their arrival. Young adult athletes could complete this history at the time of the examination while waiting in the assembly area.

The athlete moves from one examination station to the next in the order given here. Only three stations—4, 5, and 7—require a physician; if only two physicians are present, 4 and 5 could be combined in one station. A description of the stations follows.

Station 1: Blood pressure, taken by health care professional. Right arm, sitting. Values demanding repeat determinations or referral for further evaluation are:

   6 to 11 years: >125/80 mmHg (boys)   >120/75 (girls)

   12 years and older: >135/90 mmHg (boys)   >130/85 (girls)

(See Chapter 5 for more precise curves of normal blood pressure related to age.)

Station 2: Visual acuity, evaluated by health care professional. Uncorrected vision less than 20/40 requires referral for further evaluation.

Station 3: Skin-mouth-eyes, tested by physician, nurse, or athletic trainer. Examination for pustular acne, herpes, dental prosthesis, severe caries, pupil inequality, rashes, tinea pedis, and other infections.

Station 4: Chest, examined by physician. Cardiac-related history is reviewed and examination performed.

Station 5: Lymphatics, abdomen, and genitalia, examined by physician for cervical adenopathy, abdominal organomegaly, testicular abnormalities, and inguinal hernia in males, and Tanner pubic hair sexual maturity rating of both male and female adolescents competing in contact sports (Figs. 2 and 3).

Station 6: Musculoskeletal examination by physician or athletic trainer. This "two-minute orthopedic examination" (Table 4 and Figs. 4 to 15) is the most productive part of the examination after the history; it is here that an abnormality affecting athletic performance and undue risk of injury are most likely to be detected. The AAP's recommended examination form (Fig. 16) includes this musculoskeletal examination.

Station 7: Review, by a physician of the results of the various components of the history and examination, as recorded on the examination form (Figs. 1 and 16). The physician may repeat those parts of the examination reported to be abnormal or equivocal and then make the final decision about the athlete's degree of participation.

Recommendations for Participation in Competitive Sports

The most commonly used list of disqualifying conditions, published by the American Medical Association, was last revised in 1976.[5] It has become increasingly obsolete due to changes in both safety equipment and society's attitude toward the right of athletes to compete despite medical conditions that increase the risk of either sustaining injuries or aggravating preexisting medical conditions. Most sports are associated with some risk, and the physician, the athlete, and the parents must weigh whether the advantages gained by participating in athletics are worth whatever risks are involved.

To assist physicians in deciding whether athletes should be allowed to participate in particular sports, the American Academy of Pediatrics in 1988 compiled a list of recommendations for participation[6] (Appendix 1, page 261). Athletic events are divided into groups depending on degree of strenuousness and probability for collision. These groups of sports are then considered in light of medical and surgical conditions to determine whether participation would create a substantial risk of injury. Certain activities such as skiing are not inherently "contact sports," yet when competitors fall and collide with the ground, they are as much at risk as participants in the more traditional collision/contact sports; they are, therefore, included in the group called "limited contact/impact." These recommendations should only be used as a guideline; the physician's clinical judgment should remain the final arbiter in interpreting these recommendations for a specific patient.

Return to Play After Concussion or Infectious Mononucleosis

These two conditions are seen commonly in adolescent athletes and present unique problems regarding when the athlete can return to competing in a collision sport. Guidelines for the athlete who has sustained a concussion are presented in Chapter 19.

Splenic rupture, spontaneous or due to trauma, is a rare complication of infectious mononucleosis. The incidence of traumatic rupture is unknown, although infectious mononucleosis has been reported as a predisposing condition among college athletes who ruptured their spleens playing football. Although almost all cases of spontaneous rupture have occurred within 3 weeks of the onset of symptoms, a few have occurred after more than a month. However, since this is a *rare* condition, many experts recommend the following schedule for resuming activity. Light conditioning activities can begin after fever has gone and as soon as the athlete feels well enough. This is often about 3 weeks after onset. Return to full activity can begin at about 1 month, if the athlete feels able, *and if the athlete's spleen is normal in size by both palpation and percussion.*[7]

Some authors have recommended a radiologic method to confirm that splenomegaly has resolved, although this is rarely practiced. Methods suggested include an abdominal radiograph, ultrasonography, CT scan, or radionuclide scan. Such studies do not appear to be cost effective given the lack of information concerning their usefulness in this situation and the rarity of splenic rupture. If the clinician chooses to use such a method, a radionuclide liver/spleen scan is apparently the most accurate.

REFERENCES

1. Schichor A. Sports physicals: are we maximizing our opportunities? *J Adol Hlth Care*. 1989;10(5):433-434
2. Goldberg B, Saaniti A, Whitman P, Gavin M, Nicholas JA. Preparticipation sports assessment: an objective evaluation. *Pediatrics*. 1980;66:736-745
3. Thompson TR, Andrish JT, Bergfeld JA. A prospective study of preparticipation sports examinations of 2670 young athletes: methods and results. *Cleve Clin Q*. 1982;49(4):225-233
4. Clement DB, Sawchuk LL. Iron status and sports performance. *Sports Med*. 1984;1:65-74
5. American Medical Association. *Medical Evaluation of the Athlete: A Guide (revised)*. Chicago, IL: American Medical Association; 1976
6. American Academy of Pediatrics, Committee on Sports Medicine. Recommendations for participation in competitive sports. *Pediatrics*. 1988;81:737-739
7. Eichner ER. Infectious mononucleosis: recognition and management in athletes. *Phys Sportsmed*. 1987;15:61-70

Table 4. The Two-Minute Orthopedic Examination

Instructions	Points of Observation	Figure
Stand facing examiner	Acromioclavicular joints, general habitus	4
Look at ceiling, floor, over both shoulders; touch ears to shoulders	Cervical spine motion	5
Shrug shoulders (examiner resists)	Trapezius strength	6
Abduct shoulders 90° (examiner resists at 90°)	Deltoid strength	7
Full external rotation of arms	Shoulder motion	8
Flex and extend elbows	Elbow motion	9
Arms at sides, elbows 90° flexed; pronate and supinate wrists	Elbow and wrist motion	10
Spread fingers; make fist	Hand or finger motion and deformities	11
Tighten (contract) quadriceps; relax quadriceps	Symmetry and knee effusion; ankle effusion	12
"Duck walk" four steps (away from examiner with buttocks on heels)	Hip, knee, and ankle motion	12
Back to examiner	Shoulder symmetry, scoliosis	13
Knees straight, touch toes	Scoliosis, hip motion, hamstring tightness	14
Raise up on toes, raise heels	Calf symmetry, leg strength	15

SPORTS PARTICIPATION HEALTH RECORD

This evaluation is only to determine readiness for sports participation. It should not be used as a substitute for regular health maintenance exams.

NAME _____ AGE ____ (YRS) GRADE ____

ADDRESS _____ PHONE _____

SPORTS _____ DATE _____

The Health History (Part A) and Physical Examination (Part C) sections must both be completed, at least every 24 months, before sports participation. The Interim Health History section (Part B) needs to be completed at least annually.

PART A – HEALTH HISTORY:
To be completed by athlete and parent

	YES	NO
1. Have you ever had an illness that:		
a. required you to stay in the hospital?	___	___
b. lasted longer than a week?	___	___
c. caused you to miss 3 days of practice or a competition?	___	___
d. is related to allergies? (ie, hay fever, hives, asthma, insect stings)	___	___
e. required an operation?	___	___
f. is chronic? (ie, asthma, diabetes, etc)	___	___
2. Have you ever had an injury that:		
a. required you to go to an emergency room or to see a doctor?	___	___
b. required you to stay in the hospital?	___	___
c. required X-rays?	___	___
d. caused you to miss 3 days of practice or a competition?	___	___
e. required an operation?	___	___
3. Do you take any medication or pills?	___	___
4. Have any members of your family under age 50 had a heart attack, heart problem, or died unexpectedly?	___	___
5. Have you ever:		
a. been dizzy or passed out during or after exercise?	___	___
b. been unconscious or had a concussion?	___	___
6. Are you unable to run 1/2 mile (2 times around the track) without stopping?	___	___

FIG. 1. Sports Participation Health Record–History Component.

7. Do you:
   a. wear glasses or contacts?   ____ ____
   b. wear dental bridges, plates, or braces?   ____ ____
8. Have you ever had a heart murmur, high
   blood pressure, or a heart abnormality?   ____ ____
9. Do you have any allergies to any medicine?   ____ ____
10. Are you missing a kidney?   ____ ____
11. When was your last tetanus booster?   _____
12. **For Women**
    a. At what age did you experience your first
       menstrual period?_____
    b. In the last year, what is the longest time you have gone
       between periods?_____

EXPLAIN ANY "YES" ANSWERS_____
_____
_____
_____

I hereby state that, to the best of my knowledge, my answers to the
above questions are correct.

Date _____

Signature of athlete_____

Signature of parent_____

PART B – INTERIM HEALTH HISTORY
This form should be used during the interval between preparticipation
evaluations. Positive responses should prompt a physical exam.

1. Over the next 12 months, I wish to participate in the following sports:
   a. _____
   b. _____
   c. _____
   d. _____
2. Have you missed more than 3 consecutive days of participation in
   usual activities because of an injury this past year?
   Yes _____ No _____
   If yes, please indicate:
   a. Site of injury_____
   b. Type of injury_____
3. Have you missed more than 5 consecutive days of participation in
   usual activities because of an illness, or have you had a medical
   illness diagnosed that has not resolved in this past year?
   Yes _____ No _____
   If yes, please indicate:
   a. Type of illness_____

FIG. 1. (continued)

4. Have you had a seizure, concussion or been unconscious for any reason in the last year?
   Yes _____ No _____

5. Have you had surgery or been hospitalized in this past year?
   Yes _____ No _____
   If yes, please indicate:
   a. Reason for hospitalization _____
   b. Type of surgery _____

6. List all medications you are presently taking and what condition the medication is for.
   a. _____
   b. _____
   c. _____

7. Are you worried about any problem or condition at this time?
   Yes _____ No _____
   If yes, please explain: _____
   _____
   _____
   _____

I hereby state that, to the best of my knowledge, my answers to the above questions are correct.

Date _____

Signature of athlete _____

Signature of parent _____

FIG. 1. *(continued)*

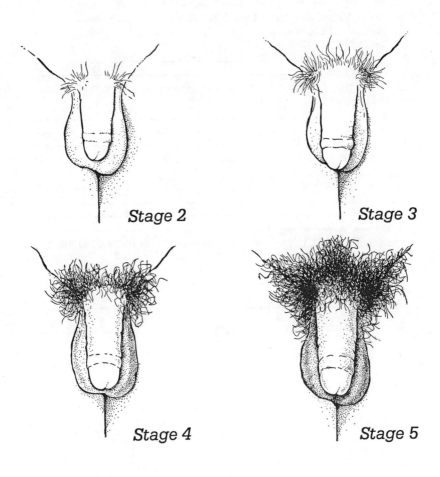

FIG. 2. Pubertal Development of Male Pubic Hair.*

Stage 2. Slightly pigmented hair laterally at the base of the penis, usually straight.

Stage 3. Hair becomes darker, coarser, begins to curl and spreads over the pubes.

Stage 4. Hair is adult in type but does not extend onto thighs.

Stage 5. Hair extends onto the thighs and frequently up the linea alba.

*Adapted from Tanner JM. *Growth of Adolescence.* 2nd ed. Oxford, England: Blackwell Scientific Publications; 1962

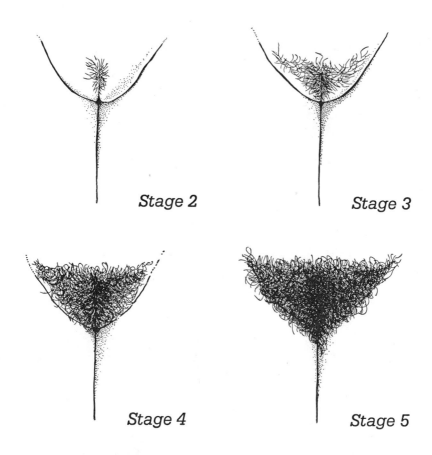

FIG. 3. Pubertal Development of Female Pubic Hair.*

Stage 2. Long, slightly pigmented, downy hair along the edges of the labia.

Stage 3. Darker, coarser, slightly curled hair spread sparsely over the mons pubis.

Stage 4. Adult type of hair but it does not extend onto thighs.

Stage 5. Adult distribution including spread along the medial aspects of the thighs.

*Adapted from Tanner JM. *Growth of Adolescence.* 2nd ed. Oxford, England: Blackwell Scientific Publications; 1962

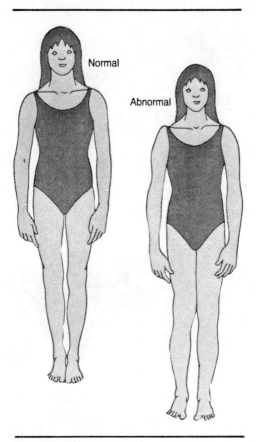

Normal

Abnormal

Stand straight with arms at sides.   **INSTRUCTIONS**

Symmetry of upper and lower extremities and trunk.   **OBSERVATIONS**
Common abnormalities:
1. Enlarged acromioclavicular joint
2. Enlarged sternoclavicular joint
3. Asymmetrical waist (leg length difference or
   scoliosis)
4. Swollen knee
5. Swollen ankle

FIG. 4.

FIGS. 4-15. The Musculoskeletal Examination.
            (Reproduced with permission of Ross Laboratories,
            Columbus, Ohio)

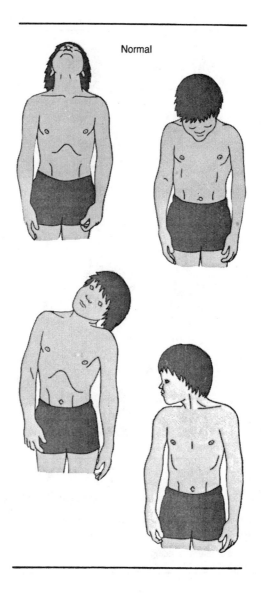

Normal

FIG. 5.

Abnormal

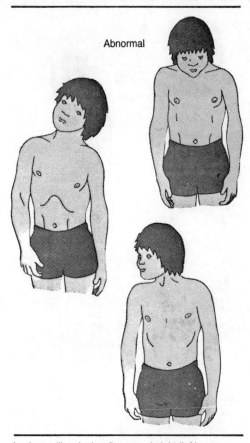

Look at ceiling; look at floor; touch right (left) ear to shoulder; look over right (left) shoulder. — **INSTRUCTIONS**

Should be able to touch chin to chest, ears to shoulders and look equally over shoulders. — **OBSERVATIONS**
Common abnormalities (may indicate previous neck injury):
1. Loss of flexion
2. Loss of lateral bending
3. Loss of rotation

FIG. 5. *(continued)*

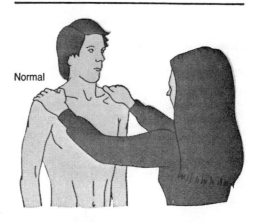

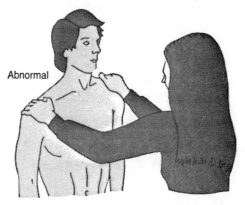

INSTRUCTIONS	Shrug shoulders while examiner holds them down.
OBSERVATIONS	Trapezius muscles appear equal; left and right sides equal strength. Common abnormalities (may indicate neck or shoulder problem): 1. Loss of strength 2. Loss of muscle bulk

FIG. 6.

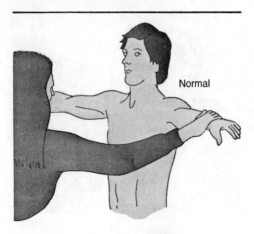

Normal

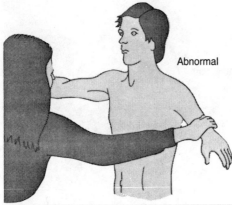

Abnormal

Hold arms out from sides horizontally and lift while examiner holds them down.

INSTRUCTIONS

Strength should be equal and deltoid muscles should be equal in size.
Common abnormalities:
1. Loss of strength
2. Wasting of deltoid muscle

OBSERVATIONS

FIG. 7.

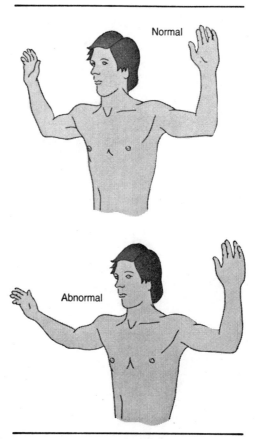

INSTRUCTIONS   Hold arms out from sides with elbows bent (90°); raise hands back vertically as far as they will go.

OBSERVATIONS   Hands go back equally and at least to upright vertical position.
Common abnormalities (may indicate shoulder problem or old dislocation):
1. Loss of external rotation

FIG. 8.

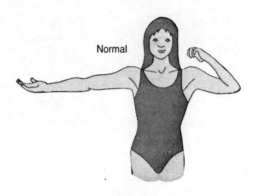

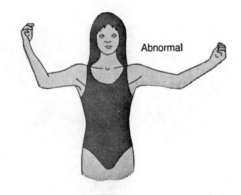

Hold arms out from sides, palms up; straighten elbows completely; bend completely.	**INSTRUCTIONS**
Motion equal left and right. Common abnormalities (may indicate old elbow injury, old dislocation, fracture, etc.): 1. Loss of extension 2. Loss of flexion	**OBSERVATIONS**

FIG. 9.

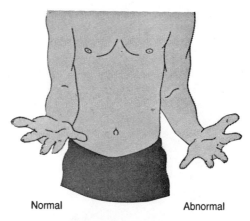

Normal   Abnormal

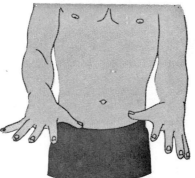

INSTRUCTIONS Hold arms down at sides with elbows bent (90°);
supinate palms; pronate palms.

OBSERVATIONS Palms should go from facing ceiling to facing floor.
Common abnormalities (may indicate old forearm,
wrist, or elbow injury):
1. Lack of full supination
2. Lack of full pronation

FIG. 10.

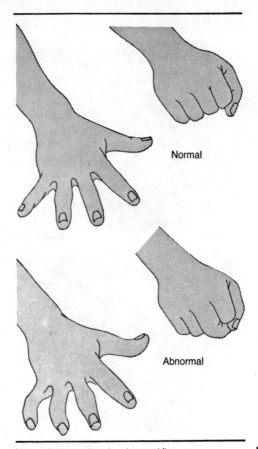

Normal

Abnormal

Make a fist; open hand and spread fingers.   **INSTRUCTIONS**

Fist should be tight and fingers straight when spread.   **OBSERVATIONS**
Common abnormalities (may indicate old finger
fractures or sprains):
1. Protruding knuckle from fist
2. Swollen and/or crooked finger

FIG. 11.

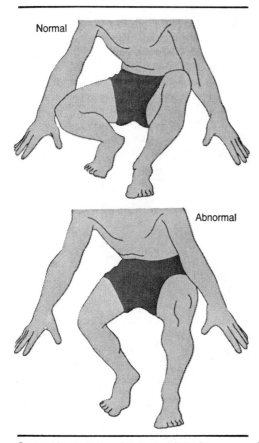

Normal

Abnormal

Squat on heels; duck walk 4 steps and stand up.	**INSTRUCTIONS**
Maneuver is painless; heel to buttock distance equal left and right; knee flexion equal during walk; rises straight up. Common abnormalities:	**OBSERVATIONS**

Common abnormalities:
1. Inability to full flex one knee
2. Inability to stand up without twisting or bending to one side

FIG. 12.

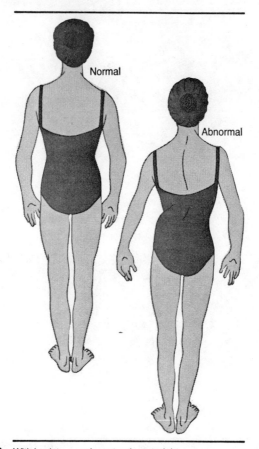

INSTRUCTIONS   With back to examiner stand up straight.

OBSERVATIONS   Symmetry of shoulders, waist, thighs, and calves.
Common abnormalities:
1. High shoulder (scoliosis) or low shoulder (muscle loss)
2. Prominent rib cage (scoliosis)
3. High hip or asymmetrical waist (leg length difference or scoliosis)
4. Small calf or thigh (weakness from old injury)

FIG. 13.

Normal

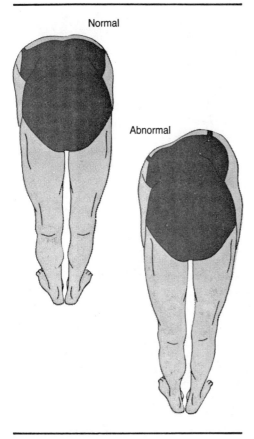

Abnormal

| Bend forward slowly as to touch toes. | **INSTRUCTIONS** |
| Bends forward straightly and smoothly. | **OBSERVATIONS** |

Common abnormalities:
1. Twists to side (low back pain)
2. Back asymmetrical (scoliosis)

FIG. 14.

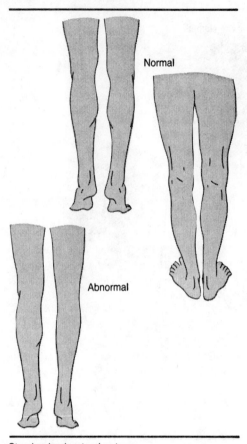

INSTRUCTIONS Stand on heels; stand on toes.

OBSERVATIONS Equal elevation right and left; symmetry of calf muscles.
Common abnormalities:
1. Wasting of calf muscles (Achilles injury or old ankle injury)

FIG. 15.

Part C – PHYSICAL EXAMINATION RECORD

NAME _____ DATE ___ / ___ / ___ AGE _____ BIRTHDATE _____

Height _____ Vision: R _____, corrected _____, uncorrected _____

Weight _____ L _____, corrected _____, uncorrected _____

Pulse _____ Blood Pressure _____ Percent Body Fat (optional) _____

	Normal	Abnormal Findings	Initials
1. Eyes			
2. Ears, Nose, Throat			
3. Mouth & Teeth			
4. Neck			
5. Cardiovascular			
6. Chest and Lungs			
7. Abdomen			
8. Skin			
9. Genitalia - Hernia (male)			
10. Musculoskeletal: ROM, strength, etc.			
a. neck			
b. spine			
c. shoulders			
d. arms/hands			
e. hips			

FIG. 16. Physical Examination Record.

f. thighs				
g. knees				
h. ankles				
i. feet				
11. Neuromuscular				
12. Physical Maturity (Tanner Stage)	1.	2.	3.	4.	5.

Comments re: Abnormal Findings: _____

_____

_____

PARTICIPATION RECOMMENDATIONS:

1. No participation in: _____

2. Limited participation in: _____

3. Requires: _____

4. Full participation in: _____

Physician Signature _____

Telephone Number _____ Address _____

American Academy of Pediatrics

FIG. 16. (continued)

CHAPTER 5

CARDIAC AND BLOOD PRESSURE EVALUATION

Heart murmurs, elevated blood pressure, and cardiac arrhythmias cause considerable concern to many physicians certifying students for competitive athletic participation.

Heart Murmur

A heart murmur may be heard in any child at some time during youth, and approximately 85% of young athletes have normal ejection-type murmurs.[1]

There may be clues in a child's history that suggest a cardiac abnormality. Three conditions–anomalous left coronary artery, mitral valve prolapse,[2] and asymmetric septal hypertrophy[3]–are often identified during adolescence. An anomalous left coronary artery, either arising from the pulmonary artery or passing between the aorta and pulmonary artery, is a rare condition that causes myocardial ischemia, which may result in angina, syncope, or sudden death. The coronary artery anomaly is frequently discovered only at the postmortem examination of an individual who died suddenly. Any child with a history of angina or recurrent syncope, particularly on exertion, should be investigated by a pediatric cardiologist because these symptoms suggest a major underlying cardiac anomaly.

Most patients with mitral valve prolapse or hypertrophic cardiomyopathy (idiopathic hypertrophic subaortic stenosis) have no symptoms. A few cases with either condition present with chest pain or arrhythmia. In both conditions a pathologic systolic murmur is usually present, which should prompt referral to a pediatric cardiologist for evaluation and recommendation regarding physical activity.

Auscultation of the heart should include assessment of rate and rhythm, systolic and diastolic murmurs, and evaluation of the heart sounds (S1, S2, and S3) and extra sounds (ejection and nonejection clicks). Particular attention should be directed toward the second heart sound (S2), listening particularly to splitting and intensity of its components. Wide, fixed splitting suggests an atrial septal defect. If a systolic ejection click is not detected, aortic valve and pulmonary valve stenosis are unlikely. Patent ductus arteriosus produces a continuous murmur, whereas aortic insufficiency causes a diastolic murmur. By means of simple auscultation, most pathologic murmurs can be detected.

Any situation increasing cardiac output also increases the intensity of both murmur and cardiac activity. Therefore, fever, anxiety, and recent exertion commonly alter the normal cardiovascular examination. If present, the youth should be reexamined when the exciting circumstances are no longer present.

When there is a definite or suspected cardiovascular abnormality, chest roentgenogram and electrocardiogram may be helpful in the evaluation. If these two studies are normal, a significant cardiovascular defect is less likely. However, a normal roentgenogram and electrocardiogram may be present in some congenital cardiac malformations, eg, mild aortic stenosis. If, after the tests, the physician continues to have concerns, he should seek consultation with a pediatric cardiologist. Any youth with a previously recognized cardiac defect should seek periodic medical clearance by a pediatric cardiologist prior to sports participation.

Many youths with congenital and rheumatic cardiac anomalies do not have hemodynamic impairment and are capable of full, active interscholastic competition. Activity guidelines for the more common cardiac malformations present in children and adolescents have been published by the American Heart Association.[4]

Blood Pressure

We concur with the Task Force[5] that made recommendations concerning hypertension in youth and techniques for measuring blood pressure. Care must be taken to obtain reliable blood pressure recordings. Some athletes have exceedingly large biceps and/or triceps, and others have long upper extremities. The width of the blood pressure bladder must be adequate to cover at least two thirds of the individual's upper arm between the top of the shoulder and the olecranon and should be of adequate length to completely encircle the circumference of the arm. The athlete should be seated at rest and the arm should be at heart level to obtain accurate readings.

Blood pressure should be measured in all youths as part of their comprehensive health maintenance. It rises continuously from birth throughout childhood, and it tends to be higher in both tall and obese children.

Charts are now available that show blood pressure ranges for American children. If a child has either a systolic or diastolic blood pressure reading above the 90th percentile (Fig. 17), the measurement should be repeated on a separate occasion. If it persists at this level after three readings, the child should be considered to have high blood pressure, and, if above the 95th percentile, as hypertensive. An algorithm for identifying, evaluating, and managing a child with elevated blood pressure is shown in Figure 18. If the child is lean, there is a possibility of an underlying cause, such as renal disease, and further investigation is needed. If the child is obese, a secondary cause is highly unlikely, but medical follow-up is necessary.

The initial treatment of children with elevated blood pressure is salt restriction, weight loss (if indicated), and exercise. Thus, participation in athletics may be beneficial to the youth with elevated blood pressure and can in fact lower diastolic blood pressure. Weight training (or "strength training") and isometric activities are not contraindicated, but weightlifting (the sport of attempting to lift a maximal weight) should be avoided.

It is rarely necessary to limit participation in athletics because of hypertension, and this should be done only after careful evaluation and consultation with a pediatric cardiologist.

Arrhythmias

Arrhythmias in children are generally caused by ectopic beats of atrial, junctional, or ventricular origin. Other less common arrhythmias are paroxysmal supraventricular tachycardia (with or without associated preexcitation syndrome), and atrioventricular block (second and third degree). A Task Force of the American College of Cardiology has made recommendations regarding arrhythmias.[6] Their conclusions are briefly summarized here.

Generally, supraventricular ectopic beats and ventricular ectopic beats have been considered benign and of little or no risk to the youngster if they are unifocal and/or disappear with exercise. Some ambiguity exists about exercise response of premature ventricular contractions (PVC). A variable response of PVCs to low-grade exercise (ie, ten sit-ups or deep knee bends) has been observed. In a few individuals, the PVCs may increase; but in most, they decrease. This variable response has been demonstrated in normal children who, when exercised intensely (heart rate greater than 140 beats per minute), had all their ectopic beats abolished.

Youths in whom ectopic beats do not disappear, or in whom there is an increase of PVCs at low-intensity exercise, should be further tested, preferably by exercise electrocardiography. If the PVCs disappear when the cardiac rate reaches 140 to 150 beats per minute, the ectopic beats are likely to be benign and do not preclude full competitive participation.

Frequent sporadic ectopic ventricular beats or those with fixed coupling (bigeminy or trigeminy) may be associated with myocarditis. Any time an ectopic rhythm occurs in a previously well child this diagnosis should be entertained. Since most children with ectopic beats are normal, the diagnosis of myocarditis should not be made on the basis of arrhythmia alone. Paroxysmal supraventricular tachycardia is not a reason for restriction from full participation if the arrhythmia can be controlled, but the advice of a pediatric cardiologist should be sought. A youth with complete heart block can lead a reasonably normal life but may be restricted in specific sports situations.

REFERENCES

1. Shaffer TE, Rose KD. Cardiac evaluation for participation in school sports. *JAMA*. 1974;228:398
2. Jeresaty RM. Mitral valve prolapse: an update. *JAMA*. 1985; 254:793-795
3. McKenna W, Deanfield J, Faruqui A, England D, Oakley C, Goodwin J. Prognosis in hypertrophic cardiomyopathy: role of age and clinical, electrocardiographic and hemodynamic features. *Am J Cardiol*. 1981;47:532-538
4. Gutgesell HP, Gessner IH, Vetter VL, Yabek SM, Norton JB Jr. Recreational and occupational recommendations for young patients with heart disease. A statement for physicians by the Committee on Congenital Cardiac Defects of the Council on Cardiovascular Disease in the Young, American Heart Association. *Circulation*. 1986; 74:1195A-1198A
5. Task Force on Blood Pressure Control in Children. Report of the Second Task Force on Blood Pressure Control in Children-1987. *Pediatrics*. 1987;79:1-25
6. Zipes DP, Cobb LA Jr, Garson A Jr, et al. Task Force VI: arrhythmias. *J Am Coll Cardiol*. 1985;6:1225-1232

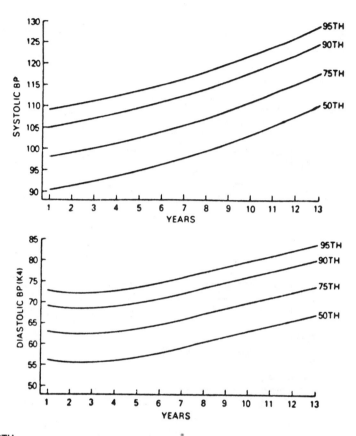

90TH PERCENTILE												
SYSTOLIC BP	106	106	107	108	109	111	112	114	115	117	119	121	124
DIASTOLIC BP	69	68	68	69	69	70	71	73	74	75	76	77	79
HEIGHT CM	80	91	100	108	115	122	129	135	141	147	153	159	165
WEIGHT KG	11	14	16	18	22	25	29	34	39	44	50	55	62

FIG. 17A. Age-specific percentiles of BP measurements in boys – 1 to 13 years of age; Korotkoff phase IV (K4) used for diastolic BP.

FIG. 17.* Age-specific Percentiles of Blood Pressure Measurements.

*From: Task Force on Blood Pressure Control in Children. Report of the second Task Force on Blood Pressure Control in Children–1987. *Pediatrics.* 1987;79:1-25 (Reprinted with permission.)

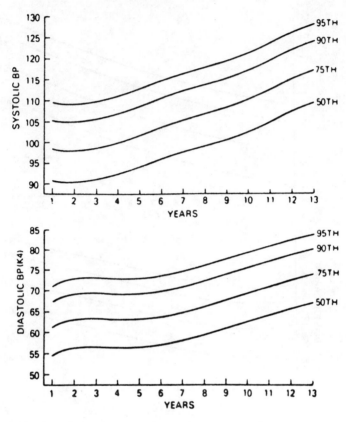

90TH PERCENTILE

SYSTOLIC BP	105	105	106	107	109	111	112	114	115	117	119	122	124
DIASTOLIC BP	67	69	69	69	69	70	71	72	74	75	77	78	80
HEIGHT CM	77	89	98	107	115	122	129	135	142	148	154	160	165
WEIGHT KG	11	13	15	18	22	25	30	35	40	45	51	58	63

FIG. 17B. Age-specific percentiles of BP measurements in girls – 1 to 13 years of age; Korotkoff phase IV (K4) used for diastolic BP.

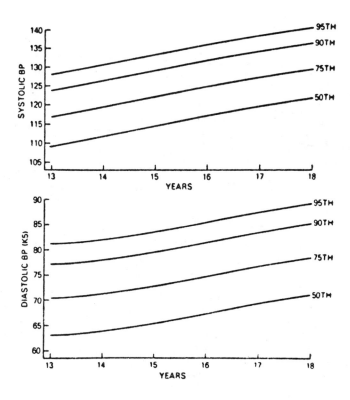

90TH PERCENTILE						
SYSTOLIC BP	124	126	129	131	134	136
DIASTOLIC BP	77	78	79	81	83	84
HEIGHT CM	165	172	178	182	184	184
WEIGHT KG	62	68	74	80	84	86

FIG. 17C. Age-specific percentiles of BP measurements in boys – 13 to 18 years of age; Korotkoff phase V (K5) used for diastolic BP.

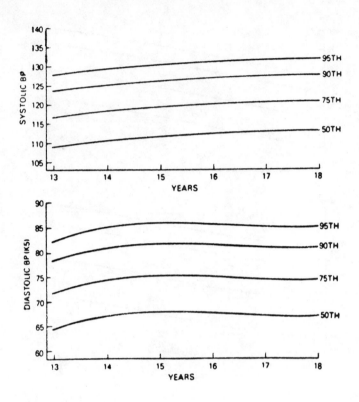

90TH PERCENTILE						
SYSTOLIC BP	124	125	126	127	127	127
DIASTOLIC BP	78	81	82	81	80	80
HEIGHT CM	165	168	169	170	170	170
WEIGHT KG	63	67	70	72	73	74

FIG. 17D. Age-specific percentiles of BP measurements in girls – 13 to 18 years of age; Korotkoff phase V (K5) used for diastolic BP.

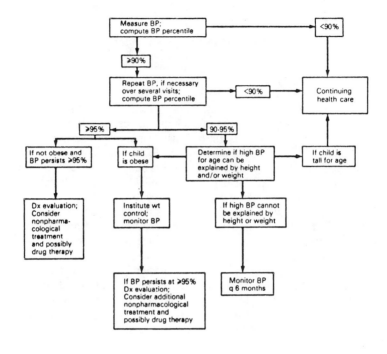

FIG. 18.* Algorithm for Identifying Children With High BP.

Note: Whenever BP measurement is stipulated, the average of at least two measurements should be used.

* From: Task Force on Blood Pressure Control in Children. Report of the second Task Force on Blood Pressure Control in Children–1987. *Pediatrics.* 1987;79:1-25 (Reprinted with permission.)

CHAPTER 6

ATHLETICS IN HOT AND COLD ENVIRONMENTS

Physical activity causes a physiologic strain to the child. Mostly taxed are the cardiovascular, respiratory, muscular, and thermoregulatory systems, which have to support an increased rate of energy metabolism. Such a strain is further magnified when exertion takes place in hot, humid, or cold environments. To maintain homeostasis on a hot humid day, the body must prevent overheating and preserve fluids. Conversely, when the child is exposed to a cold climate or to exercising in cool water, the challenge is to prevent excessive heat loss.

When the combined metabolic and climatic stresses are excessive, there may be major shifts in core body temperature and in fluid balance. These may result in decreased physical performance and compromised well-being and health. The purposes of this chapter are to review the physiologic processes that take place during exercise in the heat or cold, highlight the relative deficiencies of thermoregulation in children, list the heat- or cold-related illnesses that may take place once the thermoregulatory system is overtaxed, and finally, suggest steps to safeguard the exercising child's well-being and prevent such illnesses.

Physiologic Changes During Exercise in the Heat

During physical exertion, metabolic heat increases. Running at 10 km per hour, for example, is accompanied by a six- to eight-fold increase in energy metabolism. Exercising at maximal aerobic power will increase the metabolism 12- to 15-fold, while short-term, extremely strenuous exercise, such as sprinting, is accompanied by as much as a 30- to 40-fold increase in metabolic rate. Some 75% to 80% of such metabolism is converted into heat.

Another source of heat is the environment. Once ambient temperature exceeds skin temperature, heat flows into the body. The higher the ambient temperature, the faster the heat flow. Unless the extra metabolic and environmental heat is effectively dissipated, body core temperature will rise to levels that may induce heat-related illness, including fatal heatstroke.

The two main strategies available to the body for heat dissipation are peripheral vasodilatation and sweating. When blood flow to the skin is augmented, more heat is convected from the muscles to the skin, to be dissipated subsequently to the environment. This procedure is effective as long as skin temperature is higher than air temperature. Evaporation of sweat cools the skin and will take place at any ambient temperature. Thus, sweating is the only effective means for heat dissipation when air temperature exceeds skin temperature (which is about 30° to 32°C, or 86° to 89.6°F). Another advantage of sweating is the large quantity of heat that it can help dissipate. Evaporation of 1 L of sweat is equivalent to cooling by 2,430 kJ (580 kcal). A 10-year-old child, for example, will produce about 650 kJ of metabolic heat while playing soccer for 30 minutes. Assuming a sweating rate of 200 mL per 30 minutes (and complete evaporation), this child will achieve evaporative cooling of nearly 500 kJ. The remaining 150 kJ will be partially dissipated from the skin by convection, conduction, or radiation and partially stored in the body. Evaporation is compromised when ambient humidity is high, or when the child is overdressed (the sweat is then trapped under the clothing and cannot evaporate).

Children's Ability to Dissipate Heat

Heat Tolerance

When exposed to a high ambient temperature, children's ability to sustain exercise is lower than that of adults. This pattern has been found during controlled experiments in the laboratory[1] and during outdoor tasks.[2] There are several possible reasons for such lower heat tolerance, as summarized in Table 5 and discussed in the following sections.

Higher Metabolic Heat

When walking or running at any given speed, children use more metabolic energy (per kilogram body mass) than do adolescents or adults. The smaller the child the higher the metabolic cost. Although the causes for such a difference are not clear, its implication is that the child produces more metabolic heat than the adult, which entails a greater strain on the thermoregulatory system.

Surface Area-to-Mass Ratio

Assuming similar body proportions across ages, the smaller the body the larger the skin surface area per body mass unit. Because the rate of heat flow to and from the body depends on the surface area, children can dissipate heat faster than adults as long as ambient temperature is lower than skin temperature. If, on the other hand, air temperature exceeds skin temperature, the heat flow into the body is faster in the child, increasing the demand for heat dissipation.

Sweating Rate

Perhaps the greatest handicap that children face in their ability to dissipate heat is their low sweating rate. Although adolescents and adults can produce as much as 500 to 600 mL sweat per meter surface area per hour during exercise in the heat, prepubescents seldom produce more than 350 mL/m^2 hr of sweat.[3] The result is that children's evaporative capacity is markedly lower.

Cardiac Output

At any given metabolic level, children's cardiac output is somewhat lower than in adults.[4] Although not demonstrated experimentally, such a low cardiac output may limit the child's ability to increase skin blood flow during intense exercise in the heat, thus limiting the convection of heat to the skin.

Slow Acclimatization to Heat

When abruptly confronted with a hot climate, one needs time to acclimatize, particularly if one is expected to exert energy in the new climate. In the unacclimatized state, the individual cannot produce a sufficient amount of sweat, which results in high body temperatures and heart rate and a reduced ability to sustain exercise. Lack of acclimatization is also a most important cause of heat-related illness. Although children, like adults, do acclimatize to exercise in the heat, it takes them longer to do so. The degree of acclimatization achieved by an adult within 4 to 6 days may take the child 10 to 12 days.[5] Until fully acclimatized, the child athlete cannot be expected to perform on a par with his previous performance in the cooler environment. To prevent illness, this child should be given reduced training and allowed longer rest periods during a practice session.

Cold Tolerance of Children

Most of the information on children's response to exercise in "hostile" environments is related to climatic heat stress. Much less is known about the child's responses to cold stress, when the issue at stake is preservation of body heat. Heat loss to the environment during exposure to the cold has been more of an issue for people at rest than for people during exercise. Like adults, children produce metabolic heat at sufficient rates during moderate and intense exercise in cold air to compensate for heat lost to the environment. Furthermore, clothes worn during exercise in the cold help prevent excessive loss of body heat.

In fact, even on very cold days, metabolic heat often exceeds heat loss, which results in heat storage and a subsequent rise in body core temperature. Examples are cross-country skiing or ice hockey, during which the child, particularly if overdressed, would store heat in large amounts, as reflected by profuse sweating. Hypothermia may occur, however, when the exercise is prolonged and of a relatively mild intensity, as in mountain climbing, hiking, and snow-shoeing.

Hypothermia is more likely to develop when the child exercises in water than in air. Thermal conductivity of water is some 30-fold that of air. Heat loss from the skin to the surrounding water is therefore considerably enhanced. Here again, the large surface area-to-mass ratio of the child is a handicap, because the rate of conductive heat loss is directly related to surface area. One should further realize that the smaller and leaner the child the greater the heat loss to the water. This has been clearly shown in a study of 8- to 18-year-old girls and boys, members of a swimming club in England. They were observed while swimming, at a pace commonly used during a training session, in 20.3°C (68.5°F) water.[6] Two findings emerged: (1) although the younger children had to leave the water after some 18 to 20 minutes, the older adolescents managed to stay in the water for 30 to 33 minutes; and (2) the rate of cooling of body core was markedly faster the younger the child. In the youngest children, core temperature dropped to a staggering 34.5° to 35°C (94.1° to 95°F); in the 17- to 18-year-old girls and boys it hardly changed. It was also found that the leaner the child the faster the cooling rate.

Fluid Balance, Drinking Habits, and Hypohydration*

Exercise-Induced Hypohydration and Its Effects on Athletic Performance

Prolonged exercise, at any climate but mostly on a hot humid day, may deplete body fluids due to sweating. Sweating rate is proportional to the intensity of exertion and to the climatic heat stress. Even though children seldom produce more than 350 mL sweat per m^2 per hour, cumulative sweat loss during 3 to 4 hours of activity in the heat may induce marked hypohydration, unless accompanied by sufficient

---

*"Hypohydration" denotes a state of deficit in body fluids; "dehydration" is the actual process of incurring negative fluid balance.

drinking. The percentage decrease in plasma volume is even greater than that of total body water because during exercise plasma escapes to the interstitial space (due to the increase in intravascular hydrostatic pressure and an increase in interstitial osmotic pressure). Urine output declines during exercise, but this only partially compensates for the marked sweat loss. Other physiologic changes that result from exercise-induced dehydration include elevation of heart rate during submaximal exercise, slight reduction of stroke volume, reduction of renal plasma volume and glomerular filtration rate, partial depletion of liver glycogen, electrolyte loss (especially sodium and chloride), and reduced endurance time and mental acuity. The most important damage caused by hypohydration is a marked deficiency in one's ability to dissipate heat.

Voluntary Hypohydration

A major question is whether the exercising child knows how much to drink in order to prevent excessive dehydration. It has long been known that adults who exert for a long time underestimate the amount of fluid that they need. During a marathon race, for example, an adult may lose 5 to 6 liters (10 to 12 lb), even when liquids are provided *ad libitum*. This phenomenon has been called "voluntary hypohydration." In a study performed in Israel,[7] 10- to 12-year-old boys who exercised intermittently for 3.5 hours in a hot-dry chamber developed voluntary hypohydration at a rate similar to that found in adults. However, for a given level of hypohydration (defined as the body-fluid deficit in percentage of the euhydrated body weight), the rise in core temperature was faster in these children than in adults. This difference is potentially dangerous for the child because an excessive rise of core temperature may lead to heat-related illness, including heatstroke. Proper fluid replenishment is therefore of particular importance. This presents a major challenge to the parent, coach, teacher, and physician, all of whom must instruct the child to drink during exercise, even when not feeling thirsty.

Deliberate Fluid Loss

In addition to inadvertent dehydration, athletes–children included –sometimes deliberately induce fluid loss. This issue is discussed in Chapter 10 of this book.

Fluid and Electrolyte Replenishment

The manner by which a child replenishes sweat loss is important for maintenance of fluid and electrolyte homeostasis. The following are to

be considered:
   a. The drinking fluid should stimulate further drinking, rather than just quench the thirst.
   b. Gastric emptying to the small intestine should be fast to avoid fluid stasis and subsequent gastric distention during exercise.
   c. The total quantity of fluid intake should be as close as possible to that of fluid loss.
   d. Electrolyte and carbohydrate content should not be excessive.

Ideally, one should anticipate and predict the volume of fluid loss and replenish the fluids accordingly. As the sweating rate varies among individuals, one can best predict by measuring the losses that the child incurred on previous occasions (eg, weigh the child before and after a practice session or competition). A point often ignored is the need for the child to be fully hydrated prior to the event. During the event, fluids should be made available every 15 to 20 minutes, and the child should be encouraged to drink them even if not thirsty. Waiting until a more "practical" opportunity for drinking (eg, halftime in football) should be discouraged.

Cold drinks are preferable to tepid or warm ones because they stimulate thirst and are emptied more readily from the stomach. There are no documented adverse effects of cold drinks before, during, or after exercise, common beliefs notwithstanding.

Electrolyte concentration in children's sweat is only about half that of postpubescents.[8] Therefore, the recommended electrolyte concentration of liquids should be lower for children than for adults. The commercially available drinks are probably too concentrated. Unless proven otherwise by research, liquids for children should not exceed 5 mEq/L Na^+ (0.3g/L NaCl) and 4 mEq/L K^+. Although ingested carbohydrates may have some benefit as an energy source in prolonged exercise (45 minutes or more), they do not contribute to thermoregulation and, in concentrations of 50 g/L or more, may delay gastric emptying. A concentration of 25 g/L is probably all the child needs.

Chilled plain water is sufficient for the exercising child who eats a balanced meal and consumes salt *ad libitum*. *Water is the fluid of choice under most circumstances.* The use of salt tablets is potentially dangerous for two reasons. First, as aldosterone activity is increased with exercise, sodium is conserved by the kidney and, in fully acclimatized children, by the sweat glands. Thus, habitual exercisers who eat and drink normally may develop a positive sodium balance. And second, because sweat is markedly hypotonic (an exception is children with cystic fibrosis), body fluids become hypertonic with prolonged exercise. A disproportionate consumption of salt will increase the hypertonicity of the extracellular space and may further deplete the intracellular fluid volume. Salt tablets have been shown to irritate the gastric mucosa.

Although coating the tablets can prevent such irritation, it may interfere with the salt absorption.

Heat-Related Illness

Heat-related illnesses (also known as "heat disorders" or "heat injuries") range in severity from benign heat cramps to mild syncope to fatal heatstroke. Table 6 summarizes their classification, etiology, clinical presentation, and prevention. For treatment of these disorders, the reader should consult standard textbooks. Although not often seen in pediatric practice, these disorders have become increasingly prevalent with the increased participation of children in such sports as marathons and "fun runs."

The most important fact regarding heat-related illnesses is that they are all preventable. One should also realize that if exercise is intense and prolonged, heat illness may occur in climates that are not excessively hot. The accumulated metabolic heat and the large sweat losses can induce these disorders (including heatstroke!) even on cool but humid days.

The syndromes listed in Table 6 are seldom manifested as discrete clinical entities; but there is a definite overlap among them. For example, heat exhaustion from salt depletion may accompany exhaustion from water depletion, which, in turn, can be accompanied by syncope. Furthermore, the all-important differentiation between heat exhaustion and heatstroke is not always clear-cut (eg, profuse sweating that typically occurs with exhaustion may also be present in heatstroke). A safe policy for treatment is to assume the worst, whenever in doubt.

Children at Special Risk

Certain children, healthy or with a disease, are particularly prone to heat-related illness, as summarized in Table 7. In order to reduce the risk of heat-related illness in these children, one should appreciate the mechanisms (known or assumed) that disrupt their heat dissipation. The most common cause for such disruption is hypohydration that results from excessive sweating (as in some cyanotic congenital heart defects and fever, but also in healthy athletes who "make weight" before a wrestling or judo competition), insufficient drinking (anorexia nervosa, cystic fibrosis), diuresis (diabetes mellitus and insipidus), vomiting, and diarrhea.

Among healthy children, the most common cause of heat-related illness is insufficient acclimatization. The potential danger of this cause cannot be overemphasized. It is particularly apparent in outdoor sports, such as football, which require intense training during the summer, often before the child has had a chance to acclimatize gradually. Data based on adults suggest that a low level of aerobic fitness is another potential cause of heat-related illness in individuals who are otherwise healthy.

Obese children, adolescents, and adults, although enjoying an advantage in cold climates, are notoriously poor thermoregulators in the heat.[9] Among high school football players who die of heatstroke, most seem to be obese and unacclimatized.[10] Such individuals should be given particular attention at the start of training season.

Prevention of Heat-Related Illness

Because all heat-related illnesses are preventable, physicians who are involved with the planning or supervision of athletic events should be thoroughly familiar with the following guidelines:

1. Ensure acclimatization to exercise in the heat. Before that stage is reached, control the intensity and duration of the activities and encourage rest periods in the shade during a practice session. Remember that children acclimatize slowly and that most adverse reactions occur during the first few days of the training season.
2. Secure full hydration prior to practice sessions and competition. Fluid volume depends on the child's size. A 30-kg child, for example, can be given 250 to 350 mL fluid as late as 20 to 30 minutes prior to the event.
3. Fluids should be readily available at the site of practice or competition. Enforce periodic drinking during the event (eg, 75 to 100 mL each 20 to 25 minutes for a 30-kg child), even though the child may not feel thirsty.
4. Fluids should be chilled and flavored to stimulate thirst. Water is the drink of choice. Bear in mind, however, that on rare occasions, overzealous drinking of water may induce hyponatremia. When giving other liquids, do not exceed 0.3 g/L NaCl, 0.28 g/L KCl, and 25 g/L sugar. Fluids that contain higher caloric value may delay gastric emptying and the subsequent absorption of water from the intestines.
5. Tailor the activities to the prevailing climate. In assessing climatic heat stress, consider humidity, solar radiation, and wind—not only air temperature. Table 4 outlines the climatic conditions at which activities should be curtailed. The American Academy of Pediatrics' statement on Climatic Heat Stress and the Exercising Child (Appendix 2) includes a weather guide graph using just the air temperature and percent relative humidity to estimate when conditions are dangerous.
6. Schedule periodic rest periods in the shade during practice. This is important for adequate dissipation of heat previously accumulated.

7. Identify and screen for close observation those athletes at risk because of lack of acclimatization, poor conditioning, and diseases listed in Table 7.
8. Avoid excessive clothing, taping, or padding on hot or humid days. Ensure optimal evaporation by use of porous clothing, fitting to the skin. A hat and clothing of light color are recommended. Avoid prolonged exposure of the skin to the sun.
9. Do not hesitate to assert your authority to adjust the hours of a practice session and competition during severe climatic heat stress. Extreme heat and humidity (Table 8 and Appendix 2) are a *bona fide* reason to cancel an event.

Medical Risks of Exercising in the Cold

Etiology and Manifestations of Hypothermia

As discussed above, children's large surface-to-mass ratio and, in some cases, greater leanness, are *a priori* causes for excessive heat loss. Under certain combinations of environmental cold and exercise intensities, this may induce hypothermia (often taken as core temperature of 35°C or 95°F) and risk to their health. Although no epidemiologic data are available regarding the relative risk of children and adults for cold-related illness, one can assume that children are at least at the same risk as adults.

Prolonged activities during which hypothermia may develop include snow-shoeing, downhill and cross-country skiing (the latter less likely), skating, mountaineering, hiking, and long-distance swimming (or just staying in the water). Inadequate clothing, wetness, and exhaustion may further aggravate the heat loss. The cardiovascular, nervous, and muscular systems become progressively affected, as manifested by skin discoloration and numbness, muscle weakness, particularly in the hands, chills, marked shivering, and exhaustion. The child will appear irrational, incoherent, and, subsequently, apathetic.

Prevention of Hypothermia

Proper dry clothing is extremely important. Multilayer clothing provides better insulation than a single layer of thick material. It also allows sweat to move away from the skin to the outside. Once wet, most fabrics drastically reduce their insulative capacity. Materials such as polypropylene, when worn directly against the skin, have been found effective as insulators.

An increase in the intensity of physical activities will raise the metabolic heat and compensate partially for heat loss. One exception is when the individual is in the water, where movement may enhance the convective heat loss and bring on early exhaustion and enhanced hypothermia. When accompanying a child during cold exposures, one should be on the alert for early warning signs, as described above. Special attention should be paid to children with little subcutaneous fat, such as in anorexia. Obese individuals, on the other hand, are better insulated and can do relatively well in the cold.

For long-distance swimming, lanolin or petroleum jelly can be applied to the skin. This will markedly increase its insulative capacity. For scuba diving and other forms of submersion, a "wet suit" is effective.

REFERENCES

1. Wagner JA, Robinson S, Tzankoff SP, Marino RP. Heat tolerance and acclimatization to work in the heat in relation to age. *J Appl Physiol.* 1972;33:616-622
2. Van Beamont W. Thermoregulation in desert heat with respect to age. *Physiologist.* 1965;8:294. Abstracted
3. Bar-Or O. Temperature regulation during exercise in children and adolescents. In: Gisolfi C, Lamb DR, eds. *Perspectives in Exercise and Sport Medicine.* Indianapolis, IN: Benchmark Press; 1989:vol II;335-362
4. Godfrey S, Davies CT, Wozniak E, Barnes CA. Cardiorespiratory response to exercise in normal children. *Clin Sci.* 1971;40:419-431
5. Inbar O. *Acclimatization to dry and hot environment in young adults and children 8-10 years old.* New York, NY: Columbia University; 1978. EdD dissertation
6. Sloan RE, Keatinge WR. Cooling rates of young people swimming in cold water. *J Appl Physiol.* 1973;35:371-375
7. Bar-Or O, Dotan R, Inbar O, Rotshtein A, Zonder H. Voluntary hypohydration in 10- to 12-year-old boys. *J Appl Physiol.* 1980; 48:104-108
8. Araki T, Toda Y, Matsushita, et al. Age differences in sweating during muscular exercise. *Jpn J Phys Fitness Sports Med.* 1979; 28:239-248
9. Haymes EM, McCormick RJ, Buskirk ER. Heat tolerance of exercising lean and obese prepubertal boys. *J Appl Physiol.* 1975; 39:457-461
10. Bar-Or O. *Pediatric Sports Medicine for the Practitioner: From Physiologic Principles to Clinical Applications.* New York, NY: Springer-Verlag; 1983

Table 5. Characteristics of Children That Explain Their
Lower Heat Tolerance Than That of Adults

Typical of Children	Implications for Heat Tolerance
Higher metabolic rate during walking and running	More metabolic heat to be dissipated
Large surface area-to-mass ratio	Greater heat flow to the body when air temperature exceeds skin temperature
Lower sweating rate	Lower capacity for evaporative cooling
Lower cardiac output at any given metabolic level	Lower capacity for heat transfer from body core to the skin
Slower acclimatization to exercise in the heat	Greater risk for heat-related illness
Faster rise of core temperature during dehydration	Greater risk from heat-related illness

Table 6. Heat-Related Illnesses: Classification, Etiology, Clinical Presentation, and Prevention*

Illness	Etiology	Presenting Symptoms and Signs	Prevention
Heat cramps	Intense, prolonged exercise in heat; negative Na^+ balance	Tightening, cramps, and involuntary spasms of active muscles; somewhat low serum Na^+	Replenish salt loss; ensure acclimatization
Heat syncope	Peripheral vasodilation and pooling of blood; hypotension; hypohydration	Giddiness, syncope (mostly in an upright resting or exercising person), pallor, high T_{re}	Ensure acclimatization and fluid replenishment; reduce exertion on hot days; avoid standing motionless
Heat exhaustion (water-depletion type)	Continuous and accumulating negative water balance	Exhaustion, symptoms and signs of hypohydration, flushed skin, reduced sweating in extreme dehydration, syncope, high T_{re} hemoconcentration	Ascertain proper hydration before effort and adequate replenishment during effort, ensure acclimatization
Heat exhaustion (salt-depletion type)	Negative Na^+ balance accumulating during a few days	Exhaustion, nausea, vomiting, muscle cramps, giddiness. More insidious than the water-depletion type	Replenish electrolytes lost, based on type and duration of effort and on climate; ensure acclimatization
Heatstroke	Extreme hyperthermia leading to thermoregulatory failure; enhanced by hypohydration	Acute medical emergency that classically includes hyperpyrexia ($T_{re} \geq 41°C$), lack of sweating (not always), and neurologic deficit (disorientation, twitching, seizures, coma). Variations of the above exist.	Ensure acclimatization; identify and exclude persons at risk; adapt activities to climatic constraints

*Adapted from Buskirk ER, Grasley WC. Heat injury and conduct of athletics. In: *Physiological Aspects of Sports and Physical Fitness.* North Palm Beach, FL: Athletic Institute; 1986:49-52

Table 7. Conditions and Diseases That Predispose the Exercising Child to Heat-Related Illness

Condition or Disease	Possible Mechanism				
	Reduced Heat Convection From Core to Skin	Insufficient Sweating	Excessive Sweating	Potential Hypohydration	Other
Anorexia nervosa	X			X	Reduced subcutaneous insulation
Congenital heart disease	X		X		
Cystic fibrosis	X			X	Insufficient drinking
Diabetes (mellitus, insipidus)	X			X	
Excessive eagerness				X	High heat production
Fever	X		X	X	Regulatory insufficiency
Hypohydration	X	X (if extreme)			
Insufficient acclimatization	X	X			
Insufficient conditioning	X	X			

Malnutrition		Reduced subcutaneous insulation
Mental retardation		Insufficient drinking
Obesity		High heat production, low specific heat and surface area
Prior heat-related illness	Various (depends on illness)	
Sweating insufficiency syndromes	X	
Sympathectomy (eg, spinal injury)	X	

Table 8. Restraints on Activities at Different Levels of Heat Stress

WBGT* °C	°F	Restraints on Activities
<24	<75	All activities allowed, but be alert for prodromes of heat-related illness in prolonged events
24.0-25.9	75.0-78.6	Longer rest periods in the shade
		Enforce drinking every 15 minutes
26-29	79-84	Stop activity of unacclimatized and other persons with high risk
		Limit activities of all others (disallow long-distance races, cut down further duration of other activities)
>29	>84	Cancel all athletic activities

* WBGT = wet bulb globe temperature. This is an index of climatic heat stress that can be measured on the field by the use of a psychrometer. This apparatus, available commercially, is comprised of three thermometers. One ("wet bulb") has a wet wick around it, to monitor humidity. Another is inside a hollow black ball ("globe"), to monitor radiation. The third is a simple thermometer ("temperature"), to measure air temperature. The heat stress index is calculated as

$$WBGT = 0.7 \text{ WB temp} + 0.2 \text{ G temp} + 0.1 \text{ temp}$$

It is noteworthy that 70% of the stress is due to humidity, 20% to radiation, and only 10% to air temperature.

CHAPTER 7

NUTRITION AND THE ATHLETE

Young athletes are ripe for knowledge about nutrition because many of them believe that nutrition is an important determinant in their athletic performance. We must take advantage of this eagerness and supply these athletes with correct and practical nutritional information.

Some dietary practices and manipulations that had been considered harmless in the past are now known to cause undesirable and sometimes toxic side effects. We will review some of their uses and abuses in this chapter, as well as review current knowledge concerning the effects of nutrition on athletic performance.

Nutritional requirements are basically the same in the athletic child as in the sedentary child, except that more calories are needed by the athlete. By appropriately increasing calories in the active child, almost all other nutritional needs will be met. We will discuss the specific role of carbohydrates, fats, proteins, vitamins, and minerals. Fluid and electrolyte considerations are discussed in Chapter 6; weight control measures in Chapter 10.

The Athlete's Diet

Calorie needs in athletes vary tremendously from individual to individual, even for those participating in the same sport. One athlete may require 3,000 calories per day to maintain weight whereas another may require 6,000 calories per day. Athletes should use selections from four basic food groups to supply their daily energy needs:[1]

milk and milk products	2 servings (4 for adolescents)
meat and protein	2 servings
fruits and vegetables	4 servings
cereal and grains	4 servings

Required calories should be consumed in a minimum of three meals a day. If greater than 4,000 calories per day are needed, between meal snacking may be necessary.

The total calories of both the athlete's and the nonathlete's diet should consist of no more than 10% to 15% protein, no more than 30% fat (less than 10% saturated fats), and 55% to 65% carbohydrates.

The Role of Carbohydrates

Carbohydrates are an important energy source in the athlete for both brief, intense (anaerobic) exercise and prolonged, submaximal (aerobic) exercise. Carbohydrates may be stored in the muscle or liver as glycogen or may be circulating in the blood as glucose.

During anaerobic exercise, muscle glycogen is the primary energy source. A decline in stored muscle glycogen during repetitive strenuous training sessions can lead to chronic fatigue or what may appear to be "burn-out" (diminished interest in competing) in the athlete.

During submaximal exercise that is primarily aerobic, both glycogen and fatty acids are energy sources. The portion of energy derived from carbohydrates during this aerobic exercise depends on several factors. First, the more intense the exercise is, the higher the percentage of glycogen used. Second, a high carbohydrate diet increases the oxidation of carbohydrates for fueling subsequent exercise. Finally, endurance training results in a shift toward greater use of fat and less of glycogen during prolonged submaximal exercise.

Glycogen stores can be increased by diet. By increasing these stores, time to exhaustion can be increased[2] (Fig. 19). The type of carbohydrates consumed—complex vs. simple—is not a factor in restoring glycogen stores. The athlete needs to consume enough total calories to match energy needs. If energy needs are not met, this may compromise the ability of the body to synthesize glycogen so that even increased carbohydrate intake may not be effective in restoring glycogen stores. The repletion of energy stores needs to occur on a daily basis for training to be optimum.

Glycogen Loading

Carbohydrate loading or "supercompensation" is a form of dietary and exercise manipulation that has been found to maximally increase muscle stores of glycogen. *The competitive advantage gained from carbohydrate loading is seen only in events lasting more than 60 to 90 minutes,* ie, long endurance events in which glycogen stores may be a limiting factor such as distance running, cycling, and cross country skiing. The time to exhaustion can be increased by this method (Fig. 20). The regimen involves two phases that begin a week before the endurance competition. During the first three days, the "exhaustive phase," the athlete consumes a diet consisting of predominately fat and protein and only 100 g of carbohydrates per day. These days should also include exhaustive training. During the remaining 3 to 4 days, exercise should be dramatically curtailed, and a high carbohydrate diet (60% to 70% of total calories) should be consumed.

Even though this process maximizes glycogen storage in muscles, there are many drawbacks to glycogen loading. During the exhaustive phase, fatigue, irritability, and decreased cognitive abilities can occur due to decreased glycogen stores. Therefore, glycogen loading according to the above regimen is not advised for young children or adolescents.

There is a much safer alternative, sometimes called "overcompensation" (Fig. 21). For the 3 to 4 days before competition, minimal exercise should be performed and a high carbohydrate diet should be consumed. Beneficial increases in glycogen muscle stores result from this, although not as great as with supercompensation. Overcompensation can be used while training younger children and adolescents.

The Role of Fats

Fat is the body's most abundant energy source. One pound of endogenous fat can provide enough energy for the average person to run 30 miles! Adipose tissue is the main depot of fatty acids oxidized to support exercise. Fatty acid oxidation can contribute 50% to 60% of the energy expended during a bout of low-intensity exercise of short duration. Strenuous submaximal exercise at 60% to 80% of the VO_2max will use less fat (10% to 45% of energy expended) because this intensity precludes adequate oxygenation of muscle tissue for oxidation of fatty acids.

Endurance training increases the capacity of muscles to use fat while sparing glycogen. The adaptive response of the adipose tissue to training includes decreased mass and increased metabolic activity, and this is why aerobic exercise is a useful component of weight-reduction regimens. Regularly performed exercise prior to maturity may decrease both adipose cell size and number.[3]

Although fat is an excellent energy source, the fat content of the diet should not exceed 30% of total calories (with less than 10% of total calories as saturated fat). High fat diets have been associated with cardiovascular disease and possibly decreased endurance capacity.[4]

The Role of Protein

Proteins are not a usual energy source during exercise; proteins are used for maintenance of vital body tissues. The exact protein requirement for athletes is difficult to estimate. The required daily amount (RDA) for protein is 0.8 g/kg body weight per day. Growing youngsters in vigorous training programs might have increased requirements to as much as 1.5 g/kg body weight per day. The average American diet with 15% protein usually supplies more than this necessary amount.

Although protein deficiencies may have serious repercussions such as muscle atrophy and weakness, protein supplements can be both harmful (causing ketosis, dehydration, gout,[5] and hypercalcemia[6]) and expensive. There is no scientific evidence that consumption of protein supplements (or single amino acids such as glycine) will increase muscle mass, strength, or physical performance. Weight lifters, body builders, and other athletes should be informed that muscle size is determined by repetitive exercise and genetic potential, and it is not enhanced by excessive protein intake.

Gelatin is often promoted as a "complete" source for body building. It is derived from the collagen of animal bone and is often a major component of protein supplements. It is one of the nutritionally poorest quality proteins available, and there is little justification for its use.

Normal dietary intake of protein (10% to 15% of the total diet) is adequate in the vigorously training athlete as long as the total caloric intake is sufficient to maintain body weight. Protein supplements or amino acids should not be used.

Vitamins and Minerals

Vitamins and minerals have been touted as ergogenic aids for athletes. There is no scientific evidence that vitamin and mineral supplements help sports performance unless a nutrient deficiency exists, an infrequent occurrence in this country. Athletes who consume a normal varied diet, with enough food to meet elevated caloric requirements, will also meet their vitamin and mineral needs. Dosages of vitamins greater than recommended for normal health are of no value to the athlete.

Diets of adolescents have frequently been reported to be deficient in B vitamins, calcium, iron, and zinc. Many adolescents have poor eating habits (skipping meals, eating "fast foods" excessively). Pediatricians should attempt to teach adolescents good nutritional habits, including the values of a varied, balanced diet.

Iron

Iron is an important component in several oxygen transport compounds—hemoglobin, myoglobin, and the cytochromes. Iron deficiency with anemia significantly decreases physical performance. Whether iron deficiency without anemia actually impairs physical performance in humans is controversial.[7,8]

Athletes who are not iron deficient can develop a "pseudoanemia" ("sports anemia") from sustained and vigorous training in which there is a measurable drop in the hemoglobin.[9] During training a small increase of the RBC mass (about 18%) can develop; but a relatively greater increase is seen in the plasma volume (about 31%) causing a relative decrease in the hemoglobin concentration, hence the term "pseudoanemia." This does not appear to affect athletic performance and does not need to be treated.

If in the evaluation of an athlete, a hemoglobin is found to be 13 mg/dL or above in a male, or 11 mg/dL or above in a female, it can be considered to be normal. If the hemoglobin is below these values, and there is microcytosis, with an MCV less than 85 fL, a trial of iron therapy should be given. Ferrous sulfate, 300 mg, three times a day, is suggested with a follow-up hemoglobin obtained in 1 month. If the hemoglobin reaches normal values, the ferrous sulfate should be continued for 3 to 4 months to help replete iron body stores. If values are not normal and compliance is assured, the iron therapy should be stopped and other causes of anemia should be investigated. Marathon runners are likely to have an iron deficiency ("runner's anemia"). Its etiology is probably multifactoral, including occult gastrointestinal bleeding and an inadequate iron intake.

Those athletes at risk for iron-deficiency anemia include menstruating females, adolescents (especially during their growth spurt), and any athlete who is restricting calories. Adolescent males and menstruating females have an RDA for iron of 18 mg/day. Amenorrheic females require approximately 10 mg/day. Dieters, especially dancers, gymnasts, figure skaters, and wrestlers, often restrict calories, and, as a result, can have insufficient iron intake. A normal varied diet contains approximately 5 to 6 mg of iron for each 1,000 calories. If insufficient calories are consumed, it is very likely that insufficient iron will be consumed.

Dietary suggestions for the increase of iron and iron absorption include the following:
1. Eat sufficient calories to maintain weight.
2. Increase vitamin C foods at each meal (vitamin C increases the absorption of iron).
3. Eat breads, pastas, and cereals that are "enriched" or "fortified with iron."
4. Eat lean red meats and the dark meat of chicken and turkey. Animal protein contains iron as heme, which is the most readily absorbed in the gastrointestinal tract: 40% absorption versus 10% for nonheme iron.

Calcium

The issue of necessary dietary calcium intake has become important recently because of increased knowledge and publicity about osteoporosis in aging women. The exact etiology of osteoporosis is not known but is felt to involve several factors–nutritional (decreased calcium intake), hormonal (estrogen deficiency usually associated with amenorrhea), physical (decreased activity), and genetic. It is estimated that 25% of women older than 65 have clinically significant degrees of osteoporosis. This is a concern in the pediatric population because prevention of osteoporosis may require measures to be taken as early as the teen-age years. A calcium deficiency in the diet is common amongst adolescents. The RDA for calcium is 1200 mg/day for adolescents. Females that are not menstruating (ie, are postmenopausal or have secondary amenorrhea) may require as much as 1500 mg/day (see Chapter 3).

The best dietary sources of calcium are dairy products and dark green vegetables. Little is known about the difference in bioavailability of calcium from dietary versus supplemental sources. Calcium supplements are also inexpensive and widely available.

Nutrition Before and During Athletic Competition

Pre-event meals should be timed and composed to minimize feelings of fullness and to prevent hypoglycemia during competition. If a large meal is eaten, it should be scheduled 3 to 4 hours before competition. Lighter meals should be eaten 2 to 3 hours before competition, and liquid meals may be taken 1 to 2 hours before. All pre-event meals should be low in fat (which slows gastric emptying), low in protein (which promotes dehydration), and high in carbohydrates (60% to 70% of total calories). High carbohydrate meals are usually readily absorbed and easily digested. Pancakes and pasta are much more scientifically sound pre-game meals than the traditional beefsteak. One or two eight-ounce glasses of water help assure adequate hydration and can be taken any time before the event.

In the last hour before a competitive event, it is wise to avoid all foods and to avoid fluids with glucose or other carbohydrates. These fluids can trigger an insulin response and subsequent hypoglycemia. Insulin also suppresses mobilization of free fatty acids from adipose tissue. Both decreased levels of blood glucose and decreased availability of free fatty acids can decrease performance capacity.[4,10]

Once exercise has begun, and insulin levels are decreased in the blood (its release inhibited by the increased activity of the sympathetic nervous system), then liquid hydration with carbohydrates may be taken. Endurance athletic performance, such as in a marathon run, can be influenced by how fluid and carbohydrate intake is managed during the event. Supplying carbohydrates may delay the onset of fatigue in these events. Recently developed commercial hydration fluids (eg, Exceed[R]), containing glucose polymers and fructose, apparently do not delay gastric emptying time, as do other carbohydrates. Initial studies of such products have indicated enhanced performance in endurance athletic events, presumably because of the increased availability of exogenous carbohydrates as an energy source.[11]

Summary

Nutritional requirements in young athletes are similar to those of their sedentary counterparts, with the exception of increased caloric needs. As these increased caloric requirements are met by a balanced diet, all other requirements including protein, vitamins, and minerals will generally be met.

Coaches and parents are known to have the greatest effect on the athlete's nutritional habits. It is important to educate them so that they encourage appropriate and practical nutritional habits in our young athletes.

REFERENCES

1. Smith NJ. *Food for Sport*. Palo Alto, CA: Bull Publishing Co; 1976
2. Costill DL, Miller JM. Nutrition for endurance sport: carbohydrate and fluid balance. *Int J Sports Med*. 1980;1:2-14
3. Oscai LB, Bobirak SP, McGarr JA, Spirakis CN. Effects of exercise on adipose tissue cellularity. *Fed Proc*. 1974;33:1956-1958
4. Bergstrom J, Hermansen L, Hultman E, Saltin B. Diet, muscle glycogen and physical performance. *Acta Physiol Scand*. 1967; 71:140-150
5. Chopma JG, Forbes AL, Habicht JP. Protein in the U.S. diet. *J Am Diet Assoc*. 1978;72:253-258
6. Linkswiler HM, Zemel MB, Hegsted M, Schuette S. Protein-induced hypercalcemia. *Fed Proc*. 1981;40:2429-2433
7. Clement DB, Asmundson RC. Nutritional intake and hematological parameters in endurance runners. *Phys Sportsmed*. 1982;10(3):37-40,43
8. Pate RR, Maguire M, Van Wyk J. Dietary iron supplementation in women athletes. *Phys Sportsmed*. 1979;7(9):81-85,88
9. Eichner ER. The anemias of athletes. *Phys Sportsmed*. 1986; 14(9):122-130
10. Foster C, Costill DL, Fink WJ. Effects of pre-exercise feedings on endurance performance. *Medicine and Science in Sports*. 1979; 11(1):1-5
11. Ivy JL, Miller W, Dover L, et al. Endurance improved by ingestion of a glucose polymer supplement. *Med Sci Sports Exerc*. 1983; 15:466-471

SUGGESTED READING

Aronson V. Vitamins and minerals as ergogenic aids. *Phys Sportsmed.* 1986;14(3):209-212

Canadian Pediatric Society, Nutrition Committee. Adolescent nutrition, IV: sports and diet. *Can Med Assoc J.* 1983;129(6):552-553

Cheung S. Issues in nutrition for the school-age athlete. *J Sch Health.* 1985;55(1):35-37

Clark N. Increasing dietary iron. *Phys Sportsmed.* 1985;13(1): 131-132

Hecker AL. Nutritional conditioning for athletic competition. *Clin Sports Med.* 1984;3(3):567-582. Symposium on nutritional aspects of exercise

Hecker AL, Wheeler KB. Protein: a misunderstood nutrient for the athlete. *NSCA Journal.* 1986;7(6):28-29

Slavin JL. Calcium and healthy bones. *Phys Sportsmed.* 1985;13(9):179-181

Wheeler KB. Carbohydrates: nutritional support for optimum performance. *NSCA Journal.* 1985;7(4):56-57

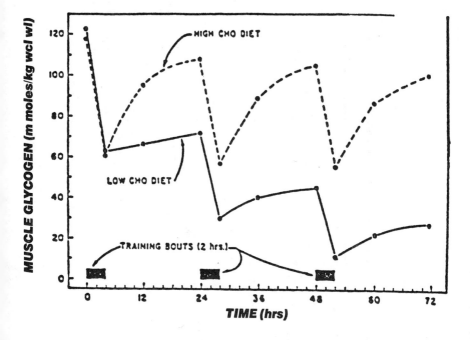

FIG. 19. Muscle Glycogen Content Is Shown During Three Successive Days of Heavy Training With Diets Whose Caloric Compositions Were Either 40% Carbohydrate (Low CHO) or 70% Carbohydrate (High CHO).

From Costil DL, Miller JM. Nutrition for endurance sports: carbohydrate and fluid balance. *Int J Sports Med.* 1980;1:2, with permission.

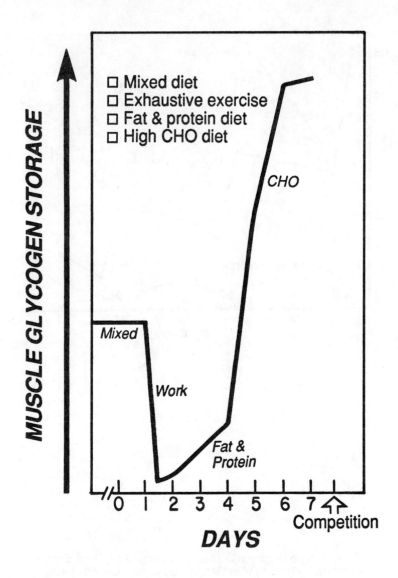

FIG. 20. "Supercompensation" Form of Glycogen-loading.

Modified from Fox EL. *Sports Physiology.* Philadelphia: WB Saunders Company; 1979, with permission.

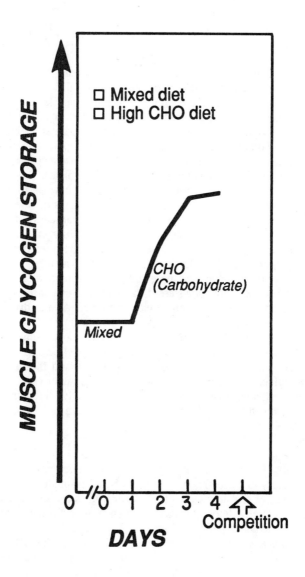

FIG. 21. "Overcompensation" Form of Glycogen-loading.

Modified with permission from Fox EL. *Sports Physiology.* Philadelphia, PA: WB Saunders Company; 1979

CHAPTER 8

STEROIDS*

Anabolic steroids (called "steroids" hereafter) have been used to enhance performance by athletes for almost three decades. Initially, they were used because of their ability to increase muscle size ("bulk-up") and hence were popular with football players who needed to increase their size and weight in order to compete successfully for line positions on a football team. Despite early scientific reports that steroids did not increase strength, and hence athletic performance, their use became widespread among nationally competitive athletes.

The initial reports indicating steroids were not performance enhancing were controlled studies using average athletes in whom continuing weight training during the period of study caused an increase in strength, regardless of whether steroids were being taken.[1] Then these studies were repeated on elite athletes who were already at their peak strength, and in whom further weight training merely kept their strength performance stable, and these athletes did increase their muscle strength in response to anabolic steroids.[2] There is no evidence that they increased aerobic capacity or endurance, however. As the drugs are considered to be carcinogenic, studies designed to further assess their toxicities or their ability to enhance athletic performance using normal volunteers as study subjects are precluded by current ethical guidelines. In 1987, the American Academy of Pediatrics reviewed the literature on steroid effects and concluded, along with the American College of Sports Medicine, that these drugs were effective in increasing muscle size, but they only increased muscle strength in elite athletes (Appendix 3).

The publicity surrounding both the decision of the National Collegiate Athletic Association (NCAA) in 1986 to begin drug testing college football players (although steroids were not among the drugs routinely tested) and the Olympic athletes being disqualified because of the presence of steroid metabolites in their urine tests has made even the most naive high school athletes aware that their performance and/or size could be enhanced pharmacologically. High school surveys in 1988 and 1989 indicated that from 6% to 11% of male adolescents were either taking them or had done so.[3,4] One third reported having begun taking them before they were 16 years of age. Surprisingly, one quarter of the users were taking them to *improve their appearance* rather than to enhance their athletic performance. The only survey that included female respondents revealed that 1.6% of high school girls acknowledged having taken them.

Anabolic steroids are derivatives of testosterone that were developed to maximize anabolic effects while minimizing the androgenic effects (Table 9). Most of the orally active steroids are produced by adding a methyl group to the C-17 alpha position of one of the basic rings of the testosterone nucleus. Most injectable steroids are esterified at the C-17 beta position. The injectable steroids are directly absorbed into the systemic circulation, and, by avoiding a first pass through the liver, are less hepatotoxic than the oral forms.

Patterns of Abuse

The list of legitimate uses of anabolic steroids is short (Table 10). Athletes abusing these drugs not only take doses 10 to 40 times greater than those prescribed medically, but they use combinations of oral and/ or injectable steroids, a practice called "stacking." By using combinations, it is hoped that although the aggregate dosage is ergogenically effective, the individual dosages will be low enough that their metabolites will be below the sensitivity threshold of a urine assay. It is also widely believed by athletes that mixtures are more effective than single drugs.

Toxic Side Effects

Youths faced with the decision of whether to take steroids should know their medical side effects (Table 11). Physicians performing individual health maintenance examinations on adolescents should consider initiating a discussion of these risks, particularly when counseling an athlete participating in a sport frequently associated with steroid use such as football, wrestling, and track and field. Team physicians not performing individual examinations should facilitate a group discussion about steroids with all of the team members early in the season.

Skeletal

Boys who take steroids in early and midpuberty, and who are still growing, can suffer premature closure of the epiphyses with resulting permanent short stature.

Cardiovascular

One of the most potentially serious consequences of prolonged use of steroids is their production of an atherogenic lipid profile, with an increase in the level of the serum low-density-lipoprotein cholesterol

(LDL-C) and an increase in the total cholesterol. This change is seen in most users, but once the steroids are stopped, these levels return to normal. Elevated blood pressure has also been reported as a side effect.

Endocrinologic

Males taking them can suffer acne, male-pattern baldness, priapism, impotence, gynecomastia, oligospermia, and testicular atrophy. Women taking them can develop hirsutism, deepening of the voice, an enlarged clitoris, and alopecia.

Hepatic

One of the most serious consequences of the prolonged use of steroids is the development of a malignant liver tumor. Another potentially fatal liver complication is the development of peliosis, a condition of multiple venous lakes within the liver that can rupture, resulting in a fatal hemorrhage. More common, but usually of less serious consequence, is hepatic dysfunction with cholestasis. The incidence of these complications is unknown.

Behavioral

Increased aggressiveness is widely believed to be a side effect, the so-called "roid rage," although objective evidence for this is inconclusive.[5] If this occurs during a collision sport such as football, then both the steroid-taking player and the player with whom he collides or fights are likely to be injured. Fortunately, most of these side effects reverse when the drugs are stopped, with the notable exceptions of peliosis, hepatoma, epiphyseal closure, and baldness in men, and the enlarged clitoris and hoarse voice in women.

What Can Be Done About It?

Steroid abuse is a serious problem, and one which is undoubtedly growing. If high school freshmen hear that most of the players on the varsity football team are taking them, then the pressures on the younger players to take them in order to make the team will be tremendous. They may not want to take them because they fear the medical side effects or because they believe it is cheating; but if they believe the only way they will be able to compete successfully for a position on the team is by taking them, then they may well make that choice. It is deplorable that young players are being put into this position.

"Drug testing" athletes is one approach to this problem, but an expensive one. Steroid assays require gas chromatography and mass spectrometry, with the cost of a single test over $100. As there are more than 1 million high school football players in the United States, this would mean more than $100 million just for one test on each player each year. Oral forms of the steroids are usually not detected by urine assay 2 to 14 days after they are last used, and even injectable steroids can be identified by assaying their metabolites only up to a month after their last use (up to a year if an oil-based formula is used). As the players are most likely to take the drugs in the spring and early summer in order to "bulk-up" prior to the season, several assays done both before and during the actual season would be necessary. Cost precludes this as a realistic solution for many school districts. (It should be mentioned that the Academy of Pediatrics in 1989 stated as a matter of policy that "athletes should not be singled out for involuntary screening for drugs of abuse," but this refers to marijuana, alcohol, etc.[6])

Coaches should address this problem at the beginning of each athletic season with a declaration that cheating in any form, including the taking of steroids, will not be tolerated. Although it is traditional for physicians not to make moral judgments about our patients' misbehavior and hence we must continue our counseling to the medical risks of steroid abuse, coaches are under no such proscription, and they can therefore declare to the athletes that *steroid use is just one more form of cheating* and therefore unacceptable behavior. We must ensure that our youth, both athletes and nonathletes, are educated about steroid side effects, and this should occur in school health classes and also during the anticipatory guidance part of the preparticipation physical examination. Unfortunately, adolescents' perception of their invincibility precludes this being very effective.

* This chapter is reprinted by permission of *Pediatrics*. Dyment PG. *Pediatrics in Review.* In press.

REFERENCES

1. Hervey GR, Hutchinson AV, Knibbs AV, et al. "Anabolic" effects of methandienone in men undergoing athletic training. *Lancet.* 1976; 2:699-702
2. Hervey GR, Knibbs AV, Burkinshaw L, et al. Effects of methandienone on the performance and body composition of men undergoing athletic training. *Clin Sci.* 1981;60:457-461
3. Johnson MD, Jay MS, Shoup B, Rickert VI. Anabolic steroid use by male adolescents. *Pediatrics.* 1989;83:921-924
4. Buckley WE, Yesalis CE, Friedl KE, Anderson WA, Streit AL, Wright JE. Estimated prevalence of anabolic steroid use among male high school seniors. *JAMA.* 1988;260:3441-3445
5. Lubell A. Does steroid abuse cause or excuse violence? *Phys Sportsmed.* 1989;17:176-180,185
6. American Academy of Pediatrics, Committee on Adolescence, Committee on Bioethics, and Provisional Committee on Substance Abuse. Screening for drugs of abuse in children and adolescents. *Pediatrics.* 1989;84:396-398

SUGGESTED READING

American College of Sports Medicine. Position statement on anabolic/androgenic steroids. *Sports Med Bull.* 1984;19:13-18

Cowart VS. Drug testing programs face snags and legal challenges. *Phys Sportsmed.* 1988;16:165-167,169-173

Dyment PG. The adolescent athlete and ergogenic aids. *J Adol Hlth Care.* 1987;8:68-73

Moore WV. Anabolic steroid use in adolescence. *JAMA.* 1988;260: 3484-3486. Editorial

Table 9. Frequently Used Anabolic Steroids

Generic Name	Trade Name	Route
boldenone undecylenate (veterinary)	Equipoise (Solvay)	injectable
methandrostenolone	called "D-ball," formerly marketed as Dianabol (Ciba)	oral
oxandrolone	Anavar (Searle)	oral
oxymetholone	Anadrol (Syntex)	oral
stanozolol	Winstrol (Winthrop)	oral, injectable
nandrolone decanoate	Deca-Durabolin (Organon)	injectable*
nandrolone phenproprionate	Durabolin (Organon)	injectable*
testosterone cypionate	Depotestosterone (Upjohn)	injectable*

* These steroids can be detected in the urine as long as a year after use, so they are not used by athletes anticipating drug testing.

Table 10. Legitimate Uses of Androgenic/Anabolic Steroids

Initiation of delayed puberty
Oxandrolone and growth hormone in Turner syndrome
Treatment of micropenis
Treatment of hypogonadism

Table 11. Anabolic Steroid Toxicities

CARDIOVASCULAR
  hypertension
  increased low-density-lipoprotein
    cholesterol
  decreased high-density-lipoprotein
    cholesterol
  increased total cholesterol

ENDOCRINOLOGIC
  acne
  male-pattern baldness
  testicular atrophy
  priapism
  impotence
  gynecomastia
  oligospermia
  decreased sperm motility
  masculinization in women

SKELETAL
  epiphyseal closure

HEPATIC
  hepatoma
  cholestatic jaundice
  peliosis

BEHAVIORAL
  aggressiveness
  increased libido
  increased energy
  irritability

CHAPTER 9

PHYSICAL FITNESS

The concept of physical fitness is understood differently by different
people and may evoke images of such diverse traits as muscular
strength, cardiopulmonary endurance, agility, flexibility, leanness, coordination, athletic success, adaptation to the heat, etc. Various activities
influence and are influenced by these traits (Table 12). The most useful
definition of fitness is that of *health-related fitness*, and it includes
optimal *muscle strength and endurance, flexibility, body composition* (ie,
degree of adiposity), and cardiopulmonary endurance. Before considering the factors that influence fitness, it is appropriate to review the
physiologic responses of children to exercise.

Responses to Exercise

Muscular work requires energy, most of which comes from adenosine
triphosphate (ATP). The ATP that enables muscle to contract can be
synthesized through either of two kinds of metabolic pathways, the
oxygen-dependent (aerobic) or the non-oxygen-dependent (anaerobic).
Aerobic work is biochemically much more efficient than anaerobic
work, with some 13 times as much substrate required to liberate a given
amount of ATP through anaerobic pathways than through aerobic. ATP
supplied anaerobically (Fig. 22) is available immediately but is
exhausted after 30 to 90 seconds. In contrast, aerobic work (Fig. 23)
must wait until local blood supply has adjusted and adequate oxygen is
available; once begun, aerobic work can be sustained for many minutes
or even hours.

Muscle fibers have a degree of specialization: some contract mostly
anaerobically and are different histochemically from those that contract
mostly aerobically. The fiber types are often referred to in functional
(as opposed to biochemical) terms, so anaerobically contracting fibers
are referred to as fast-twitch; aerobically contracting fibers are called
slow-twitch or fatigue-resistant. Explosive exercise, such as jumping,
throwing, or sprinting, depends heavily on fast-twitch (anaerobic)
fibers; endurance events like the marathon rely almost entirely on abundance of slow-twitch fibers (Fig. 24). Many activities (mile run, soccer,
etc.) that have elements of both continuous movement and high-
intensity, quick bursts of action require a mixture of slow- and fast-
twitch fibers.

It is not clear what determines an individual's distribution of fibers.

Adult elite athletes in sprint and throwing events have a roughly even mix of slow- and fast-twitch fibers, whereas successful marathoners have a preponderance of slow-twitch, and it has been suggested but not demonstrated that this distribution is genetically determined. The influence of training on fiber-type distribution will be discussed later in this chapter.

One more distinction between aerobic and anaerobic work is important: During anaerobic exercise, lactic acid is produced; this is not the case for aerobic work. Lactic acid must be buffered to prevent systemic acidosis: as part of this buffering process, carbon dioxide is produced, creating an extra ventilatory load for the respiratory system to eliminate.

Responses to Increasing Workloads

During a single session of exercise that involves increasing intensity, the body responds in many ways, most importantly related to delivery of oxygen to the exercising muscles and elimination of carbon dioxide from those muscles.

Cardiovascular Responses

In order to oxygenate more blood, and to deliver more oxygenated blood to exercising muscles, cardiac output must increase some fivefold from rest to a maximum attainable workload. The greater cardiac output is made up by increases in both stroke volume and heart rate (Fig. 25). In the absence of heart block or drug therapy, maximal heart rate depends on age. For children and adolescents, it is 195 to 215 beats per minute. Cardiac stroke volume depends heavily on fitness and is readily increased by conditioning. Cardiac output is usually one of the important factors limiting exercise tolerance in healthy children (and adults) and in those with heart disease. Systolic blood pressure increases during rhythmic exercise by as much as 100 mm Hg in healthy adolescents. Diastolic blood pressure remains unchanged. In contrast, during static exercise (so-called "isometrics," where a muscle is contracted steadily but no movement takes place), both systolic and diastolic blood pressure rise, sometimes abruptly. Despite the increased blood pressure, oxygen uptake and delivery do not increase during static exercise. Therefore, myocardial oxygen demand is increased (to accomplish the work implied by the increased blood pressure), yet myocardial oxygen supply is not increased. In most healthy children and adolescents, this increased blood pressure does not present a danger.

Ventilatory Responses

Like the cardiac pump, the ventilatory pump increases its output considerably in the transition from rest to maximum exercise. During exhausting exercise, minute ventilation may be as high as 10 to 15 times the resting value. Also similar to the output of the cardiac pump, the ventilatory apparatus increases its output by increases in both the size of the individual strokes (tidal volume) and their frequency (respiratory rate) (Fig. 26). Tidal volume can increase to about 50% of vital capacity, whereas maximal respiratory frequency is roughly 70 breaths/minute for healthy 5-year-olds and 50 breaths/minute for healthy teen-agers. Ventilatory capacity never limits exercise tolerance in children with normal lungs. In fact, minute ventilation during maximum exercise seldom exceeds 50% to 70% of a child's resting maximum voluntary ventilation (MVV).

Muscle Metabolic Responses

As more oxygenated blood is delivered to the exercising muscles, the oxygen must be processed by mitochondrial enzymes to liberate ATP. The oxidative capacity of muscle, along with a finite cardiac output, is usually an important factor in limiting exercise tolerance. Muscle mitochondrial density, and, therefore, oxidative capacity, can be increased with conditioning.

Maximal Oxygen Consumption (VO$_2$max)

The greatest volume of oxygen that the exercising subject can take in and process during a progressively difficult exercise test is termed the maximal oxygen consumption (VO$_2$max). This is the variable most often selected by physiologists to represent a person's aerobic fitness. VO$_2$max depends on the links in the oxygen delivery chain already discussed and can be limited by the weakest link in the chain (Fig. 27). If oxygen cannot be brought into the body and transferred to the blood (respiratory system), delivered to the exercising muscles (cardiovascular system), or processed by the muscle mitochondria (muscle metabolic system), VO$_2$max will be low, and aerobic exercise capacity will be proportionately low. The person will be relatively unfit.

Anaerobic capacity is also an important component of overall fitness. Anaerobic capacity depends on the presence of fast-twitch muscle fibers, the availability of the enzymes needed for anaerobic glycolysis such as phosphofructokinase, ATPase, creatine kinase, and the ability of the muscles to tolerate high lactic acid concentrations. Like aerobic fitness, anaerobic capacity is influenced by both genetic endowment and training.

Body Composition

Adiposity is determined by a fairly straightforward balance equation: calories *in* (diet) minus calories *out* (energy expended through basal metabolism, growth, a small amount lost in the stool, and physical activity). Contrary to popular belief, *many obese children have lower caloric intake than their lean peers.* This points to the calories-out portion of the equation as the more important one. In children as well as adults, underactivity is associated with obesity, from infancy onward. Extra body weight may lead to reduced activity, but persuasive evidence from animals and human children indicates that the relationship may also be in the other direction, namely underactivity *causing* obesity.

Body composition is as relevant to success in competitive athletics as it is to general health. The extra weight that a cross-country runner with 20% body fat has to carry will put him or her at a disadvantage in competition with a runner with a lower percentage of body fat. However, minimal weight is not a reasonable or helpful goal. For example, the wrestler who has dieted and sweated and urinated off 5 pounds will also be at a disadvantage in a match with an opponent who is the same weight without resorting to debilitating rituals.

Flexibility

The ease and extent to which body parts can progress actively or passively through their range of motion is called flexibility, an important part of fitness. In competitive athletics, where frequent near-maximal exertion (during competition or training) causes micro tears or mini tears of muscles and tendons, flexibility is often lost. This loss of flexibility comes about as the result of the fibrosis that is a normal part of the tissue repair process. Stiff muscles, tendons, and joints are at greater risk for injury than flexible tissues. Therefore, without careful attention to flexibility, a young, highly motivated athlete can become trapped in a cycle of injury and reinjury.

Relationship Between Fitness and Health

It would seem logical that fitness would improve longevity. Yet despite some suggestive epidemiologic studies, no unequivocal advantage has been demonstrated for fit individuals over the unfit in terms of life expectancy.

It is an equally compelling notion that fitness should prevent various diseases, but again the data are scarce. Several advantages have been demonstrated for active people compared with those who are less active, yet it is not clear that aerobic fitness itself is essential for these advantages. That is, some epidemiologic studies in adults indicate that *activity*, and not necessarily cardiovascular fitness, is associated with decreased risk of disease; the activity may be of an intensity that is too low to increase VO_2max, yet may confer other advantages. Several risk factors for cardiovascular disease are favorably affected by increased levels of activity, including increased levels of high-density lipoprotein (HDL) cholesterol, the protective fraction of cholesterol; lowered levels of triglycerides; decreased obesity; and (often) less smoking. Activity seems to help prevent osteoporosis in postmenopausal women. There are no data to suggest that an active or fit person is less likely than the average sedentary person to develop pulmonary problems (except through decreased smoking), acute infectious diseases, metabolic diseases, or cancer.

There *have* been some clearly identified benefits of fitness and activity for patients already suffering from various chronic illnesses. These will be discussed in Chapter 20.

Factors Influencing Fitness

Maximal aerobic power is determined by several factors, including heredity and the amount and intensity of habitual activity. The more sedentary a person, the more unfit. One study of trained athletes showed a dramatic loss of cardiopulmonary fitness after only three weeks of bedrest and demonstrated the recovery of fitness with an exercise conditioning program thereafter. What is seen in three weeks of absolute bedrest is almost certainly seen with extended periods of relative inactivity.

Conditioning

Several of the links in the fitness chain can be strengthened with conditioning programs. Given the appropriate frequency, intensity, and duration of exercise, VO_2max can definitely increase. There is still some controversy about whether children can increase their aerobic fitness (VO_2max) to the degree that adults can, but few disagree that most children can experience some improvement in fitness.

Specificity of Training

The type of fitness or the type of activity one wishes to improve through a conditioning program will determine the type of conditioning stimulus that must be used because of the principle of specificity of training. This means that if the goal is to improve leg muscle endurance, one must do leg exercise. More generally, if one wishes to improve aerobic capacity, one must use aerobic exercise in the training program. If one wishes to increase anaerobic capacity, then anaerobic exercise must be repeated.

Frequency of Exercise for Increasing Aerobic Fitness

Aerobic capacity is increased most dependably with exercise sessions at least three to five times each week. Fewer sessions may have some effect; more frequent sessions (every day) may have a slight additional positive effect, but at the cost of increased likelihood of injuries, especially in a weight-bearing activity like jogging.

If the goal of the training program is improved athletic performance, training frequency (and duration and intensity) will of course be greater than the frequency required for fitness alone.

Intensity of Exercise for Increasing Aerobic Fitness

Exercise intense enough to require 70% to 85% of a person's VO_2max will be sufficient to increase that maximum, if it is repeated long enough and frequently enough. This intensity is usually associated with heart rates of about 90% of maximum. For healthy children and adolescents, this translates to a heart rate of 150 or more beats/minute. Recent evidence suggests that even less intense exercise may suffice for increasing aerobic fitness, especially in subjects who begin with low fitness levels.

Duration of Exercise for Increasing Aerobic Fitness

Exercise sessions must last at least 15 minutes, and the program of three to five weekly sessions must last 6 weeks or longer to increase fitness. Many unfit individuals may have difficulty exercising (for example, jogging) at the target intensity for 15 minutes on their first try, but may tolerate 5 or 10 minutes comfortably. Even children with severe disabilities are very often able to increase their tolerance of exercise sessions if they start very gradually. Some successful programs have started with 10 minutes per session during the first week, and have added 2 to the exercise session each week. By this progression, children who were just barely able to tolerate 10 minutes of light exercise at a time have been able to exercise continuously for 30 minutes within 10 weeks. If the goal is a lifelong program, it clearly is worth the time needed to increase duration.

Type of Exercise for Increasing Aerobic Fitness

For increasing aerobic capacity, the preceding guidelines for the frequency, intensity, and duration of exercise should be carried out with aerobic exercise. Aerobic exercise is exercise of submaximal intensity, which uses large muscle groups and is done rhythmically, repeatedly, and continuously. Brisk walking, jogging, swimming, bike riding, cross-country skiing, rowing, etc., all qualify as aerobic exercise. Stop-and-go activities, such as racquet sports, football, lifting heavy weights, etc., are not aerobic.

Increasing Flexibility

Some of a person's flexibility is determined by genetic factors and some by unalterable structural factors; however, flexibility *can* be improved, especially with a good stretching program. Stretching can be done regularly and is most effective (and safest) when done when the muscles are warm. Therefore, a morning jogger should probably not attempt extensive stretching before the run, but rather after a few minutes of easy jogging have warmed the muscles. The most effective stretching is actually done *after* the run. The two main kinds of stretching are static and ballistic. In a static stretch, the muscle is stretched gradually, with prolonged force applied in a single direction. A ballistic stretch uses body weight and gravity or momentum to stretch a muscle. This is a bouncing kind of manuever and carries with it the danger of overstretching the muscle, thereby tearing it. Ballistic stretching should be discouraged.

Anaerobic Conditioning: Increasing Muscle Strength and Power

There are many instances where the goal is not simply increased aerobic capacity or improved cardiopulmonary fitness. Instances where improvements in specific aspects of anaerobic fitness are sought are especially common in preadolescents and adolescents, particularly in those involved in competitive athletics. In these instances, the goals are increased muscle strength (as opposed to endurance) and/or bulk (and definition) of specific muscle groups.

Strength training (also called "weight training") with "free weights" (weight systems including the time-honored barbells where the weights are not part of a fixed apparatus) or with one of the multistation apparatus like Nautilus or Universal has been popular for some time among adolescents, with the Nautilus/Universal type increasing in popularity tremendously in the last 5 years. These programs involve making parts of the body move through given ranges against varying resistances. For example, one might sit on a bench and perform knee flexions, pulling downward with the heel against an adjustable amount of weight via a pulley system. This form of exercise can in fact be very successful in increasing skeletal muscle strength, even in prepubertal children.

The principles behind these training programs include specificity, increasing resistance, and alternating stress and rest. Specificity simply requires triceps exercise to increase triceps strength; leg lifts will not increase arm strength. Increasing resistance implies that the untrained muscle will be able to move relatively small weights or resistances; beginning a program with attempts at moving maximum weight will only induce injury. Instead, a program should begin with the athlete performing tasks that can be easily accomplished; once it is clear that recovery occurs after a training session, it should fairly quickly increase to more challenging loads. Strength will not improve unless the load is at least 60% of the maximum weight the athlete can lift in a single effort. As strength increases, the training load will also need to increase to provide continued improvement. Alternating stress and rest is required for the muscle to repair micro tears that accompany any stressful training session and to build new muscle. In some cases this will require a rest of several days; in other cases, several hours will be enough time between workouts.

During performance of weight lifting exercises, heart rate and blood pressure typically increase with proportionally little increase in oxygen consumption (although this may be less true in children than in adults). This means that there is an increase in myocardial oxygen demand which is out of proportion with the increase in oxygen supply. In most healthy children and adults, this discrepancy presents no threat to health. Therefore, in most adolescents, strength training (weight training) will not only enhance athletic performance but may also improve the self-image of a youngster who has seen himself or herself as skinny and weak. These programs should supplement, not replace, aerobic programs because they do not influence cardiopulmonary fitness.

Habitual Activity

Obviously, exercise sessions need not be designed as part of a formal program to have their effect. In the first years of life, most children are active enough to maintain moderately good aerobic capacity, without supervised, prescribed exercise programs. However, this does not seem to hold true into the elementary school years or beyond, and relative inactivity is a common pattern among healthy children and adults in industrialized nations. Acute and chronic illnesses often add further to inactivity. Television has probably had the largest single influence on children's play and exercise time in recent decades. In fact, television now accounts for some 25 hours in the week of a typical North American child. It is ironic that the habit of activity is as unpracticed as it is, given the high degree of interest in sports in our society. A Canadian study of 10- to 12-year-old children revealed that they spent 12 hours each week watching televised sports programs, yet less than 3 hours per week participating in vigorous activity.

To blame decreased levels of childhood fitness on television alone would be an oversimplification, and one that ignores the important contribution of family (ie, adult) factors. Data from other fields may be relevant here: it is quite clear that patterns set or witnessed in the formative years have a powerful influence on subsequent adult behavior. Children of smokers are much more likely to smoke as adults than children of nonsmokers. Similarly with exercise, it makes sense to assume that children introduced early to the example of an active life style would be more likely to adopt it as their own than those who never see that choice.

Physiologic Changes with Conditioning

Aerobic conditioning programs produce several changes which enable more oxygen to be consumed and, therefore, more aerobic exercise to be performed (Table 13).

Changes in the Cardiovascular System

Maximum cardiac output increases after conditioning. Maximum heart rate does not change, and continues to depend only on age. Therefore, the other component of cardiac output—stroke volume—must (and does) increase, at least in postpubertal adolescents and adults. This increase can range from 10% to nearly 50% of preconditioning values. Increased stroke volume means that a similar cardiac output (and oxygen delivery) can be accomplished at a lower heart rate, and, in fact, lower resting heart rate is a hallmark of the fit state.

Changes in Ventilation

No significant changes occur in the lungs with conditioning. Minute ventilation at maximal exercise is greater than before conditioning, but this is only because nonventilatory factors, which had limited exercise before conditioning, have improved, exercise can proceed further, and the ventilatory demands of the new higher exercise loads must be met. The ventilation at maximal workloads is still less than 70% of the resting maximal voluntary ventilation (MVV), and the MVV has not increased.

Changes in Muscle Metabolism

Through aerobic conditioning, skeletal muscle can increase its aerobic capacity, a change reflected histochemically by increased mitochondrial density. It is not known whether endurance training can actually alter the distribution between slow- and fast-twitch fiber type. Anaerobic training increases the activity of enzymes involved with anaerobic metabolic processes, while little affecting oxidative enzyme activity.

Testing

Pediatricians are sometimes interested in evaluating the habitual activity or fitness of individual children or groups of children to assess the effects of physical education programs or to compare baseline fitness or activity levels with those of comparable children.

Assessing Habitual Activity

Numerous tools exist for estimating the level of habitual activity in children, ranging from direct one-on-one observation, to recall methods (questionnaires that ask about activities during the preceding days or weeks), to electronic monitors that measure various components of activity (impact, changes in posture, changes in heart rate, etc.). None of these methods is perfect, but each has advantages.

Fitness Testing

Direct measurement of oxygen uptake is very expensive in terms of equipment, trained personnel, and time. In some cases it is well worth the investment; however, there are several more broadly applicable tools that measure some of the components of fitness. The most widely used in the past few decades in the United States has been the test sponsored by the President's Council on Physical Fitness and Sports. This instrument consists of a battery of seven tests, including sit-ups, pull-ups, standing long jump, shuttle run, 600-yard run, and softball throw for distance. National standards are well established for these tests. Students who score in the top percentiles in these tests are given a Presidential Fitness Certificate. Unfortunately, none of the items on the test measures fitness in a way that is meaningful to health, but rather they are tests of skill, agility, or explosive strength. Therefore, what the President's Council rewards is athletic ability and not fitness. The large child who has matured early is rewarded, and the small child is penalized.

The American Alliance for Health, Physical Education, Recreation, and Dance (AAHPERD) has established a testing system that has received widespread use for several years and goes a long way towards correcting the deficiencies in the older test. The AAHPERD Health-Related Fitness Test includes tests of endurance fitness (a 1-mile run or a 9-minute run for distance, the choice being at the discretion of local authorities), body composition (skinfold fat measurement), flexibility of the low back (a "sit and reach" test), and abdominal muscle strength and endurance (sit-ups). Perhaps most importantly, the "superstars" are not rewarded, nor are the less endowed penalized by omission from awards ceremonies; in fact, guidelines are included for remedial work for students who fall below the 20th percentile, so they may improve. At the time of this writing, the AAHPERD Health-Related Physical Fitness Test seems to be the best mass testing system available for children.

Fitness Testing in the Physician's Office

Several tools for assessing fitness can be used in the physician's office. Increasing numbers of commercially available computer-driven "metabolic carts" allow actual measurement of maximal oxygen consumption. However, these systems are very expensive, require sophisticated technical support, and, therefore, are not useful for most office settings. A fairly inexpensive cycle ergometer or portable step, together with a heart rate monitor, can permit valuable office-based fitness testing. In the healthy child, maximal power output (highest workload achieved) on a cycle ergometer during a protocol using progressively increasing workloads is nearly as informative as maximal oxygen consumption.

Physical working capacity at a heart rate of 170 beats per minute (PWC 170) is also a frequently used measurement, which avoids the difficulties of determining whether a true maximal effort has been put forth and also avoids the subject fatigue necessitated by a maximal effort.

Power output can be estimated for a step test wherein a child ascends and descends a 30-cm step at 15 times per minute for 5 minutes, then 22.5 times per minute for another 5 minutes, and then at 30 times per minute for a final 5 minutes.

Power (watts) = Body weight (kg) $\times$ 3.92 $\times$ N/60
where N = number of steps per minute.

This equation should be calculated for each workload for which you want to know the power output. In most cases, this will only be the highest workload.

Other step tests use the heart rate in the recovery period after the stepping task.

Table 12. Typical Effects of Various Sports on Components of Fitness*

Type of Sport	General Stamina	Local Muscular Endurance	Muscle Strength	Speed	Agility	Flexibility	Body Weight Control
Individual sports							
Boxing	+++	+++	++	+++	+++	–	+++
Cycling (long and middle distances)	+++	+++	++	++	–	–	+++
Figure skating	++	+++	++	+	++	+++	++
Golf	–	–	+	+	–	++	++
Gymnastics	+	+++	+++	++	++	+++	++
Horseback riding	–	++	+	–	–	–	–
Jumping (track and field)	+	+	+++	+++	+	+++	+
Rowing	+++	+++	+++	+	–	+	+++
Running							
sprint	+	+	+++	+++	++	+	+
middle distances	+++	+++	++	++	+	+	+++
long distances	+++	+	+	+	–	–	+++
Sailing	+	+++	++	+	++	–	+
Skiing							
downhill/slalom	++	+++	++	++	+++	+	+
cross country	+++	++	++	+	+	–	+++

* – = Hardly any effect, + = some effect, + + = much, + + + = very much.

Table 12. Typical Effects of Various Sports on Components of Fitness* *(continued)*

Type of Sport	General Stamina	Local Muscular Endurance	Muscle Strength	Speed	Agility	Flexibility	Body Weight Control
Swimming	+++	+++	++	++	+	++	+++
Tennis (squash)	++	++	++	++	+++	+	++
Throwing (discus, etc)	+	++	+++	+++	++	++	+
Walking	++	+	+	−	−	−	++
Weightlifting	−	++	+++	+++	+	+	+
Wrestling, judo	++	+++	+++	++	++	+++	++
Team sports							
Baseball	+	++	+	++	++	+	+
Basketball, soccer	++	++	+	++	++	+	++
Football (American)	++	+++	+++	+++	+++	+	++
Ice hockey	++	+++	++	+++	+++	+	++
Volleyball	+	++	++	++	+	++	+
Water polo	+++	+++	++	+	+	++	++

* − = Hardly any effect, + = some effect, ++ = much, +++ = very much.

Table 13. Physiologic Effects of Conditioning

Function	Effect
Cardiac	
Heart rate	
Maximum	no change
Submaximum (including rest)	decreases
Stroke volume (rest and exercise)	increases
Maximum cardiac output	increases
Pulmonary	
Resting pulmonary function	no change
Maximum exercise ventilation	increases
Muscle metabolic	
Mitochondrial density	increases
Oxidative enzyme activity	increases

ANAEROBIC METABOLISM

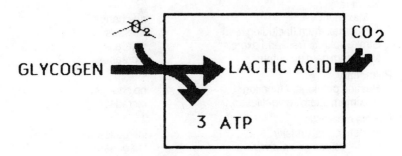

FIG. 22. Schematic of anaerobic metabolism (ie, inadequate oxygen supply) at the mitochondrial membrane, for the same arbitrary amount of glycogen, showing much lower energy yield and higher carbon dioxide production necessitated by buffering lactic acid formed.

AEROBIC METABOLISM

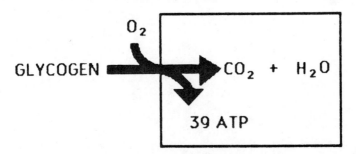

FIG. 23. Schematic of aerobic metabolism (ie, adequate oxygen supply) at the mitochondrial membrane for an arbitrary amount of glycogen.

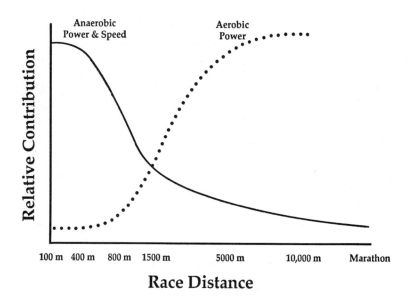

Race Distance

FIG. 24. Relative contributions of aerobic and anaerobic power for various competitive running events from 100 meters to 42.2 km, showing increasing contribution of aerobic and decreasing contribution of anaerobic power.

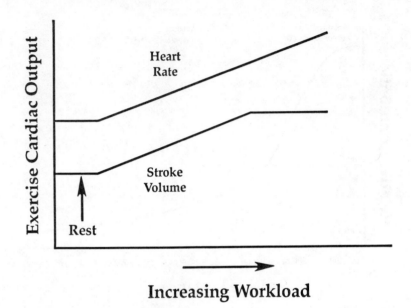

FIG. 25. Cardiac Responses to Increasing Workloads.

As workload increases, so too does cardiac output in order to supply more oxygen to, and remove carbon dioxide from, the exercising muscle. Cardiac output increases first through increases in both stroke volume and heart rate, until stroke volume plateaus at a point that depends largely on the individual's aerobic fitness. When stroke volume can no longer increase, further increases in cardiac output come through increased heart rate alone.

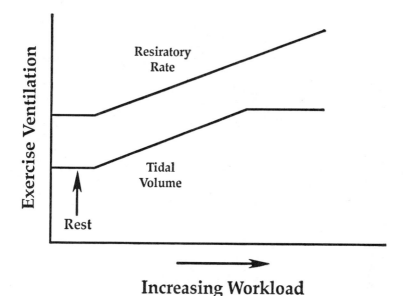

FIG. 26. Ventilatory Adjustments to Increasing Workloads.

As workload increases, total minute ventilation also increases in order to remove metabolically produced carbon dioxide and to supply oxygen. The increases in ventilation are made up by increases in both tidal volume (bigger breaths) and respiratory rate (more breaths), until tidal volume reaches roughly 50% of resting vital capacity. Further increases in minute ventilation are then produced by increases in respiratory rate alone.

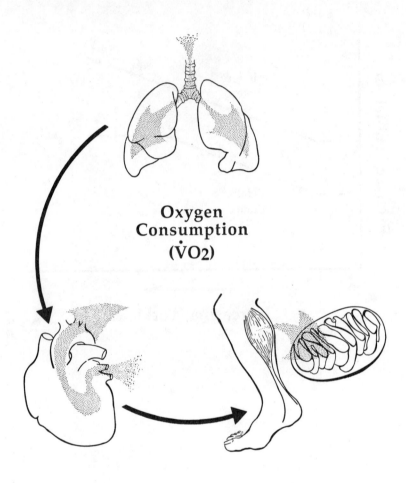

Oxygen Consumption ($\dot{V}O_2$)

FIG. 27. Links in the Oxygen-supply Chain.

Oxygen enters the body via the lungs, where it is loaded onto hemoglobin; it is then delivered to exercising muscle by the cardiovascular system; it is finally processed in the muscle mitochondria in a process that produces energy and muscle contraction.

CHAPTER 10

WEIGHT CONTROL IN ATHLETES

Weight control issues affect virtually all sports. Athletes involved in sports emphasizing power are often faced with the problem of enhancing lean body mass by balancing exercise and increased nutritional needs. Conversely, wrestlers are often required to limit nutrient intake in order to lose weight for competition in lower weight classes. Basketball players who have tremendous aerobic energy expenditure often require huge daily caloric intake, whereas gymnasts and ballet dancers often starve themselves to maintain thinness. The physician advising these athletes needs a variety of skills to adequately provide counseling regarding weight control.

Understanding the methods of assessing and interpreting body composition and applying them to specific athletes and sports is important. Unfortunately, the optimal body composition has been validated for very few sports. Although average percent body fat of participants in many sports has been demonstrated, the significance related to performance and health is unclear.

Assessment of Percent Body Fat

The use of ideal height/weight charts for determining ideal weight should be a thing of the past. Underwater weighing, skin fat fold measurements, and impedance measurements are all methods that are either accepted or being developed. However, the proper use of these techniques is still being debated.[1]

Underwater weighing has long been the "gold standard" for assessing body fat. Even with the use of this valuable tool, varied techniques have led to conflicting results. The availability of underwater weighing equipment is limited. Recent attempts to use impedance measurements to determine percent body fat have not yet proven reliable.

The most widely used and simplest tool for determining percent body fat is the *skin fold caliper*. Plastic skin fold calipers are readily available from medical supply houses. They are as accurate as more expensive models but are not as durable. Lange skin fold calipers are made of metal and are quite durable and accurate. Several manufacturers make computerized calipers that calculate the body fat composition automatically. Plastic calipers are perfectly acceptable for routine use.

In skilled hands, skin fold measurement error using calipers is ± 3%. Larger errors might occur in measurements taken by unskilled examiners. Percent body fat determinations using calipers are based on certain assumptions regarding underlying lean body mass.[1] The standards in this chapter were developed from data on adult males.[2] However, athletes in different sports may have different bone densities and amounts of body water. Individual variations in lean mass density and body water may skew the results of calculations.

Technique

A variety of calculations using measured skin folds in different parts of the body have been developed. The Jackson-Pollack formula,[2] using the sum of three skin fold measurements, has been shown to be as accurate as sampling more sites.[3] To use this formula, begin by taking three skin fold measurements.

Use of Skin Fold Calipers

If right handed:
1. Hold caliper in right hand.
2. Firmly grasp a "pinch" of two layers of skin and all the underlying fat with thumb and forefinger of left hand. Do not pick up underlying muscle.
3. Place caliper jaws one-half inch from fingers at a depth about equal to the thickness of the fold.
4. Release the caliper jaws.
5. Read the dial to the closest 0.5 millimeter. Read within 2 seconds.
6. Procedure may be repeated 3 times to increase accuracy.
7. Anatomic sites for measurement (Jackson-Pollack formula)

   Chest: A diagonal fold one third of the distance between the anterior axillary line (front-most level of the armpit) and the nipple

   Abdomen: A vertical fold 1 inch to the side of the umbilicus.

   Thigh: With weight supported on the nondominant leg and the knee of the dominant leg slightly bent. A vertical fold on the front of the thigh (dominant leg) halfway between the hip and knee.

The sum of these measurements is then used to determine the current percent body fat of the wrestler by referring to Table 14. An alternative method for determining percent body fat involves more complex calculations that would best be performed on a computer. This equation, developed for and validated on high school wrestlers, is as follows[6]:

Percent body fat = (1.48 × chest sf) + (.075 × subscapular sf) + (.077 × triceps sf) + (.160 × suprailiac sf) + (.102 × thigh sf) + (.152 × abdominal sf)

sf = skin fold measurement

The athlete should be advised as to what ideal wrestling weight to maintain for competition. Many an athlete's wrestling weight has been determined by what other wrestlers are available to compete for the team in particular weight categories. In the 1970s, recommendations for ideal minimum percent body fat emanated from the Iowa wrestling studies. Most successful wrestlers compete with 5% to 7% body fat.[4] It is assumed that this percentage of fat was adequate to ensure health and normal growth and development. More recently and disturbingly, an increasing trend of elite wrestlers competing with less than 5% body fat has been revealed from the Iowa Wrestling Studies.[5]

Percent body fat determinations should be performed during the pre-participation examination well before the season starts because the athlete needs sufficient time to lose weight safely. The method to calculate the ideal wrestling weight (ie, 6% body fat) is given in Table 15.

Ideally, a team physician should be working with not only the athletes but coaches, school administrators, parents, and, if present, a certified athletic trainer to develop standards for all the wrestlers at the school. Some school systems have adopted programs setting minimal percent body fat at which any wrestler may compete.

Direct physician involvement with the wrestling program may have more impact than counseling the individual athlete. Rule changes for the sport of wrestling could lessen the need for athletes to reduce to unrealistic weights in order to meet team needs. By changing rules to allow more wrestling weight categories, particularly for the smaller athletes, or if more than one athlete were allowed to compete at the same weight, the practice of fitting wrestlers to weight categories might be curtailed.

Coaches and athletes need to be convinced that starvation, sweating techniques (such as use of saunas or exercising in rubber suits), and diuretic or cathartic use have no place in the management of weight loss. Dehydration produces an acute loss of strength and endurance that cannot be regained in the short time between weigh-in and competition. If an athlete repeatedly dehydrates (a practice called "bouncing"), the accumulated effect on stamina and strength may reduce performance in the latter part of the season.[5]

Weight Reduction Guidelines

Ideal wrestling weight determinations should be made well in advance of the beginning of the season. The athlete should be allowed enough time to "make" his wrestling weight without having to lose more than 2 lbs per week. On occasion (particularly when football players need to lose weight for wrestling season), a weight loss program designed to lose 4 lbs per week may be permissible for short periods of time.

The average adolescent male at the time of peak height velocity may require 2,500 to 3,000 kcal/day to maintain normal growth. No adolescent athlete should drop below an intake of 2,000 kcal/day. Table 16 contains some hints for the wrestler who must diet and exercise to reduce to an ideal wrestling weight.[7,8]

A program that will result in an intake of approximately 2,000 kcal/day is presented in Table 17. More complex calorie counting programs are not necessary. Calorie reductions greater than this may actually result in the cessation of growth for the adolescent.

It takes approximately a 3,500-kcal deficit to lose 1 lb of fat. Because of differing metabolic rates, the averages will not apply to everyone. Some athletes may become discouraged if progress is not monitored and adjustments made in the program.

If the athlete is to lose 2 lbs per week, a 1,000-kcal/day deficit is required. Based on the above dietary considerations, decreased calorie intake could account for 50% of the deficit. The remainder must consist of increased calorie expenditure through an emphasis on aerobic exercise. Exercises such as running, swimming, bicycling, racquetball, and even circuit training with weights (ie, rapid interval station work with high repetitions and low weights) are appropriate.

Table 18 presents some exercise activities and their caloric expenditure equivalents. It is important to emphasize that the caloric expenditures listed are for activities done by individuals of average body weight, with the exception of weight lifting where size does not influence the amount of calories expended.

If the average-sized athlete restricts his/her diet by 500 kcal/day and expends another 500 kcal/day by increasing exercise (ie, running 3 miles/day [300 kcal] plus 20 minutes of circuit weight training [200 kcal]), a weight loss of 2 lbs/week could be expected. It is important to remember individual differences and to monitor the athlete's progress in order to make adjustments in his/her weight loss program.

Weight Gain Guidelines

Ethical considerations in advising the athlete who wants to gain weight in excess of normal growth are significant. The long-term health consequences to the cardiovascular system of the athlete who wants to build greater muscle bulk are probably detrimental. What happens to that athlete after he completes his competitive years? Theoretically, the stresses placed on the skeletal system of supporting excess weight and power generated by larger than normal muscle mass may contribute to excessive injury rates. However, the football player who has been told by his coach to gain 20 lbs over the summer is highly motivated. It is unlikely that the physician will be able to dissuade him. Proper counseling will at least help ensure the safest practices to gain weight.

The use of anabolic steroids to increase body size ("bulk-up") is mentioned only to be condemned (see Chapter 8). Protein supplements in the form of powders and pills are very expensive and are most often very poorly bioavailable (many are made from cattle horns and hooves). Excess protein intake may add to the acid load on the body, which may potentially reduce endurance capacity for the athlete. Protein is also the worst energy source for the athlete who needs to consume what may be enormous numbers of calories. A growing athlete needs only about a half gram of protein for each pound of body weight, an amount usually exceeded in the diet of typical American teen-agers.[9,10]

It is important that the athlete's diet contain a proper balance of the basic food groups. In the off season, the adolescent's diet should contain at least four servings per day of the dairy, fruit-vegetable, and grain groups, and two servings from the meat group. During the training season there should be at least eight servings per day from the fruit-vegetable and grain groups, four servings from the dairy group, and two from the meat group.[9,10]

Assuming that 3,500 kcal is approximately equivalent to 1 lb of weight, the athlete will need to consume 1,000 kcal/day above his usual metabolic requirements in order to gain 2 lbs/week. In the athlete who may already require 4,000 kcal/day to maintain weight, the consumption of an additional 1,000 kcal may be difficult. It is virtually impossible to consume that amount of kcal in a totally balanced diet and still have time to go to school and participate in his sport. Once the individual has assured adequate intake of nutrients with frequent balanced meals, the source of excess calories becomes less important. Intake of high-calorie-dense snacks may be appropriate. Useful products may include puddings and drinks designed to provide balanced nutrients and approximately 375 kcal per serving. They have the advantage of being well balanced and easily consumed. Candy and chips may also have a role in boosting the athlete's caloric intake.

Distinct from weight loss programs, weight gain programs should emphasize anaerobic strength and muscle building exercises. If the athlete increases aerobic exercise, the gains of increased caloric intake will be lost. Strength training with weights is probably the best method of ensuring that the weight gains produce increased lean body mass rather than fat. An athlete should not try to lift weights every day. A one-day rest between workouts will allow time for recovery and growth (see Chapter 9).

As is the case with weight loss programs, frequent monitoring and adjustments will be necessary. The athlete may become easily discouraged and frustrated if he is told only that he will have to consume 3,500 kcal/week in addition to his regular intake in order to gain 1 lb. Increasing weight beyond usual gains is an extremely difficult and expensive task to perform during an adolescent's period of rapid growth.

REFERENCES

1. Wilmore JH. Body composition in sport and exercise: directions for future research. *Med Sci Sports Exerc*. 1983;15(1):21-31
2. Jackson A, Pollack M. Practical assessment of body composition. *Phys Sportsmed*. 1985;13(5):76-90
3. Thorland WG, Johnson GO, Tharp GO, Fagot TG, Hammer RW. Validity of anthropometric equations for the estimation of body density in adolescent athletes. *Med Sci Sports Exerc*. 1984;16(1):77-81
4. Tipton CM, Tcheng TK. Iowa wrestling study: weight loss in high school students. *JAMA*. 1970;214(7):1269-1274
5. Tipton CM, Oppliger RA. Iowa wrestling study: lessons for physicians. *Iowa Med*. 1984;74:381-385
6. Wilmore J. Body composition and athletic performance. In: Haskell W, Scolla J, Whittam J, eds. *Nutrition and Athletic Performance*. Palo Alto, CA: Bull Publishing Co; 1982:158-175
7. Smith N, Massuco BA. *Nutrition: Food for sport*. Seattle, WA: Division of Sports Medicine, University of Washington School of Medicine
8. Smith N, Masuco BA. *A weight control program for the high school wrestler*. Seattle, WA: Division of Sports Medicine, University of Washington School of Medicine
9. American Academy of Pediatrics, Committee on Nutrition. *Pediatric Nutrition Handbook*. Elk Grove Village, IL: American Academy of Pediatrics; 1985
10. *Food Power: A coaches' guide to improving performance*. Rosemont, IL: National Dairy Council; 1983

SUGGESTED READING

Smith NJ, Worthington-Roberts B. *Food for Sport*. 2nd ed. Palo Alto, CA: Bull Publishing Company; 1989

Table 14. Percent Fat Estimates in Adolescent Males, Using Three Skin Fold Determinations*

Sum of Skin Folds (chest, abdomen, thigh)	Percent Fat
11-13	2.2
14-16	3.2
17-19	4.2
20-22	5.1
23-25	6.1
26-28	7.0
29-31	8.0
32-34	8.9
35-37	9.8
38-40	10.7
41-43	11.6
44-46	12.5
47-49	13.4
50-52	14.3
53-55	15.1
56-58	16.0
59-61	16.9
62-64	17.6
65-67	18.5
68-70	19.3
71-73	20.1
74-76	20.9
77-79	21.7
80-82	22.4
83-85	23.2
86-88	24.0

*From Jackson and Pollack[2]; reprinted with permission of McGraw-Hill, Inc.

Table 15. Method to Calculate Ideal Wrestling Weight

$$\text{Desired Weight} = \frac{\text{weight} - [\text{weight} \times \% \text{ fat}/100]}{1 - x}$$

x = desired % body fat in decimal form

Example

Assume: current wt. = 150

current % fat = 10.7%

desired % fat = 6%

$$\text{Desired wt.} = \frac{150 - [150 \times 10.7/100]}{1 - .06}$$

Desired wt. = 142 lbs.

Table 16. Dietary Advice for the Wrestler Trying to Lose Weight*

---

1. Eat three meals a day.
2. Eat what is normally served at home.
3. Take smaller portions than usual.
4. Avoid fatty foods (chips, butter, cheese, mayonnaise).
5. Give up desserts.
6. Use skim milk and diet soft drinks.
7. Avoid all between-meal snacks (snack foods are loaded with fat and sugar).
8. Don't talk about your diet or weight problem. It's your problem and don't make it a family affair.
9. Don't weigh yourself more often than once a week.
10. If you feel hungry, drink water.

---

*Reprinted by permission of Nathan J. Smith, M.D.

Table 17. Sample 2,000-Calorie Diet*

Meal	Amount	Calories
BREAKFAST		
Fruit	1 serving	100
Bread group	2 servings	250
LUNCH		
Sandwich, hamburger, or cheeseburger	1 serving	400
French fries	20 pieces	230
Milk	1 pint	170
DINNER		
Meat	6 ounces	450
Medium potato	1 each	80
Vegetable	1 serving	40
Roll and butter	1 serving	125
Milk	1 pint	170

*Reproduced by permission of Nathan J. Smith, M.D.

Table 18. Calorie Expenditure of Different Activities

Activity	Calories Expended
Running	100 kcal/mile
Swimming	1200 kcal/hr
Racquetball	900 kcal/hr
Basketball	900 kcal/hr
Bicycling (12 mph)	600-900 kcal/hr
Circuit weights	500-600 kcal/hr

CHAPTER 11

EPIDEMIOLOGY AND PREVENTION
OF SPORTS INJURIES

Thirty million children and young adults between the ages of 6 and 21 engage in out-of-school sports programs. Three and one half million boys and almost 2 million girls participate in interscholastic sports.[1] With these large numbers of sports participants, it is essential that the pediatrician be aware of the potential health problems that young athletes may incur. Sports injuries, an integral part of sports participation, is an obvious area for epidemiologic investigation.

Epidemiologic studies in sports medicine are performed to determine the distribution or rate of health problems, most often injuries, that result from athletic participation. This information identifies the risk of participating in a selected sport and allows the young athlete and his parents to decide if they wish to assume this injury risk. It also permits for the planning of necessary medical coverage, provides for the anticipation of the occurrence of specific injuries, and allows for the surveillance and comparison of individual programs and sports. Additionally, epidemiologic studies can identify significant variables that are related to the occurrence of an injury and may suggest causal relationships. This information can be used to design studies to modify those factors associated with injury and thereby optimally reduce injury rates through preventive intervention.[2]

Epidemiologic studies in sports medicine have employed various methodologies.[3,4] Case studies generally review a series of patients seeking medical care for an injury or a series of specific injuries in a specific sport. These studies provide descriptive information, but they cannot establish a measure of risk. This is because they lack a defined "exposed" population that potentially could be injured, such as all members of a team or a league or all participants at a specific event. Studies that provide an "at risk" population can make observations concerning the frequency of specific injuries and make correlations between the chance of being injured with select variables. Data are accumulated retrospectively, by identifying those previously injured; prospectively, by following a group of athletes prior to their injury; or by a combination of both methodologies.

Epidemiologic studies in sports medicine have encountered many problems. These include the inaccurate reporting of injuries, the lack of consistent definitions of injury, the unavailability of true athletic exposure times, the use of unique and thereby select populations, the lack of a consistent grading of the severity of injury, the inability to control variables, and the lack of funding. These problems, often unsolvable because of the unique circumstances of athletic competition, have made it difficult to establish accurate, broad generalizations about children's athletic experiences, to compare different experiences, and to draw etiologic relationships. Despite these limitations, the epidemiologic studies in the last 30 years have provided important information about the injury experiences of children and have suggested specific factors that may be associated with injury. The remainder of this chapter will focus on the results of these studies and will provide the pediatrician with the necessary information to discuss the risks of participation and to recognize the areas for potential preventive intervention.

General Studies

Several studies have been performed to review the general sports injury experiences of children. DeHaven,[5] in a case study at a sports medicine specialty clinic, found that 12% of all visits during the study period were for children under 15 years of age. Of these children, 71% were between 14 and 15, and males presented three times as often as females. The most common injuries were sprains and strains (25%), followed by fractures (20%) and patellofemoral syndrome (16.1%). The lower extremity accounted for 69% of the injuries, and the upper extremity 26%. Football had the most injuries of any sport (38%), followed by basketball (11.1%) and soccer (9%).

Zaricznyj et al[6] studied school-aged children in Springfield, IL, and found that 6% each year sustained traumatic sports injuries requiring at least first aid. Three percent of all elementary, 7% of junior high school, and 11% of high school children were injured. Males sustained 67% of the injuries. Fourteen-year-old girls and 15-year-old boys were most likely to be injured. Forty percent of the injuries occurred in nonorganized sports, 38% in physical education class, 15% in organized school sports, and 7% in community programs. Football was associated with the highest injury rate, followed by basketball, gym games, baseball, and roller skating. The head was most often injured (19.6%), followed by the fingers (18.9%), ankle (11.4%), and knee (10.6%). Only 20% of the injuries were considered serious.

Gallagher et al[7] studied 87,000 children in Massachusetts. An overall injury rate of 22.4% was found, with a sports injury rate of .15% for children less than 5 years of age, 3.4% for 6- to 12-year-olds, and 7.03% for 13- to 19-year-olds. No deaths were related to sports. Sports injuries represented the most common cause of injury for the 13- to 19-year-olds and overall was the second leading cause of emergency room visits and hospital admissions. Sports injuries were also the leading cause of fractures (other than skull) and sprains. The largest proportion of injuries resulted from football (19.9%), basketball (17.4%), rollerskating (13.4%), and baseball (9.4%).

Garrick and Requa[8] evaluated 3,049 interscholastic athletes for sports-related medical problems that required removal from participation. An overall injury rate of 39% was found, but 73% of the injuries required less than 5 days of restriction. The sports with the highest injury rates per 100 participants for boys were football (81), wrestling (75), track and field (33), basketball (31), soccer (30), and cross-country (30); for girls, softball (44), gymnastics (40), track and field (35), cross-country (35), basketball (25), and volleyball (10).

The above studies (Table 19) demonstrate that between 3% and 20% of children engaged in sports activities are injured per year and approximately three quarters of these injuries are minor. Adolescents sustain a greater number of injuries than do younger children. Younger children appear to be most often injured during nonorganized sports activities; adolescents sustain most injuries in competitive organized sports.

Studies have been performed to compare the injury experiences of males and females. Shively et al[9] found similar rates of injury in basketball, baseball, and track and field, but higher rates for males in cross-country and for females in soccer and swimming. Garrick and Requa[8] also found similar injury rates in basketball and track and field, but a higher rate of female injuries in gymnastics. Chandy and Grana,[10] conversely, found no differences in the frequency of swimming or cross-country injuries, but a higher rate of female injuries in basketball. Males appear to sustain a greater relative percentage of shoulder injuries; females appear to be relatively more susceptible to knee and ankle injuries, to overuse injuries, and to injuries that require surgical correction.[9,10]

These general studies provide an overview of the injury experiences of children in sports. Specific sports present unique demands and risks, and the injury experiences of children participating in the more popular sports merit discussion (Table 20).

Baseball

Baseball is a sport that exposes participants to both macrotraumatic collision injuries and microtraumatic overuse problems. The former occur from collisions either with the ground, the ball, or another player, and the latter from repetitive throwing. "Little League elbow" has received the most attention. Adams,[11] in 1965, reported a 45% incidence of elbow pain among 9- to 14-year-old pitchers, with symptoms most often localized to the area of the medial epicondyle. Radiographic studies of a sample demonstrated either hypertrophy of the humerus, medial epicondylar epiphyseal fragmentation and separation, or osteochondrosis of the capitellum and radial head. The presence of these radiographic findings and the frequency of the symptoms raised great concern for the potential of a chronic elbow disability resulting from ultimately aseptic necrosis, osteochondritis dissecans, and/or chronic arthritis. Recommendations for limitations on the amount of pitching and for restrictions on curve balls in Little League followed. Ten years later, Gugenheim et al[12] and Larson et al[13] studied groups of young pitchers and found only a 17% to 20% incidence of symptoms, with a 10% to 12% incidence of flexion contractures and a 3% to 37% occurrence of valgus deformity. Although radiographic abnormalities were identified, the incidence, apart from humeral hypertrophy, was much lower than in the study by Adams,[11] and Gugenheim et al and Larson et al were unable to correlate radiographic abnormalities with symptoms. Most importantly, they found no cases of aseptic necrosis of the capitellum or radial head and were unable to correlate pathology with the amount of pitching experience.

Torg et al[14] evaluated a less structured and competitive baseball league in which only limited restriction was placed on the amount of pitching, and curve balls were permitted. Although 70% of the pitchers reported symptoms, radiographic evidence of significant pathology was not observed. The author suggested that the pressure to pitch despite symptoms of pain eventually might lead to more significant pathology.

The effect of early pitching on the eventual development of a chronic disability of the elbow or shoulder remains to be completely established. "Little League shoulder" represents fracture of the proximal humeral epiphyseal plate and is not as common as elbow abnormalities. A long-term follow-up of young pitchers by Francis et al[15] determined that 13% still had elbow symptoms but significant residual damage was rare. For young players who continue, or begin, to pitch during adolescence, the risk of developing significant musculoskeletal pathology has been demonstrated. Grana and Raskin[16] noted a 4% incidence of loose bodies at the elbow in a group of adolescent pitchers, and Barnes and Tullos[17] described ulnar friction spurs with ulnar nerve symptoms, muscle ruptures, medial collateral ligament ruptures, loose bodies, and degenerative arthritis in collegiate and professional pitchers. It remains to be determined whether pitching in the preadolescent years predisposes to these problems or if these more significant pathologic processes only result from the greater forces generated by older and stronger adolescents and young adults.

The overall incidence of baseball injuries occurring in preadolescent players appears to be low, but studies are limited. Hale,[18] in an internal organizational study of Little League baseball, reported a 2% injury rate; most often injured were batters (22%), runners (17%), catchers (16%), and outfielders (14%). Most injuries were to the head (38%) and upper extremities (37%), with contusions (40%), fractures (19%), and sprains (18%) being the most common types of injury. Most injuries occurred when players were hit by a pitched ball (22%), hit by a batted ball (19%), catching (14%), hit by a thrown ball (10%), or sliding (10%). At the high school level, Garrick and Requa[8] found an injury rate of 18%, and Shively et al[9] a rate of 14%.

A rare injury that is unique to baseball is cardiac damage and arrhythmia secondary to nonpenetrating chest trauma from a batted or pitched ball.[19] Twenty-three deaths were recorded in 5- to 14- year-olds between 1973 and 1981. A suggestion has been made for chest pads to be worn by batters and pitchers.

Football

Football is a collision sport where the risk of injury arises mainly from the forces generated at the time of contact. Epidemiologic studies of the sport have demonstrated that the injury experience is significantly related to the level of competition, with preadolescent injuries decidedly different from those seen in high school and college. This may well be related to the intensity of the forces generated at the time of contact. As force is directly related to mass and velocity, faster and heavier participants would be expected to sustain more significant injuries.

Children 8 to 14 years of age have been shown to have an overall injury rate of between 15% and 20%.[20,21] Using the National Athletic Injury Reporting System (NAIRS) classification of injury, Goldberg et al[22] found a 10% rate of significant injury per season (significant injuries are those requiring more than 7 days of restriction from participation). Younger players in the lower division of youth football sustained significantly fewer injuries than older children playing in the higher division. Fractures, sprains, contusions, and strains were the most common injuries. The hand/wrist, knee, shoulder/humerus, and ankle/foot were most often injured, and the upper body accounted for almost 50% of the injuries. Quarterbacks/runningbacks, defensive linemen, offensive linemen, and linebackers were the players at greatest risk for injury. Injuries that could create a permanent musculoskeletal disability were rare, and cervical neck injuries resulting in paralysis were not reported. Epiphyseal fractures accounted for 3% of the injuries, and all in the study responded to medical management. Surgical intervention for the treatment of injuries was rare. Variables that appeared to be related to the risk of injury included larger size in the oldest division, pile-ups after the play was completed, reinjury of an incompletely resolved prior injury, and impact with the helmet. An adult responsible for the surveillance of injuries was found to be a needed addition to the supervisory staff.

High school football injuries present a very different injury experience. The NAIRS study[23] revealed a total injury rate of 64% and a significant injury rate of 16%. Moretz et al[24] found an overall injury rate of 25% and a 12% rate of significant injuries, and Blyth and Mueller[25] found a 48% injury rate, 17% of which were significant. At the high school level, significant sprains and strains were most common and were decidedly more prevalent than in youth football where fractures were the most common significant injury. Additionally, the lower extremity, particularly the knee and ankle, were most likely to be injured; in younger competitors it was the upper extremity. Knee injuries account for 15% to 20% of all injuries, approximately 92,000 annually. Four percent of injured high school football players required surgical intervention, which projects to approximately 14,380 cases per year in the United States.[26] Knee injuries accounted for 69% of this total. Runningbacks, defensive linemen, and linebackers were most likely to be injured. A greater number of injuries occurred in practice than in games, but, if corrected to numbers of injury per exposure (ie, game or practice), the games were associated with eight times the frequency of injury.

Specific variables that correlate with likelihood of injury at the high school level include older age, heavier weight, varsity-level competition, greater number of years of experience, and prior injury. Additionally, improved field surface conditions, a limited contact program, and the use of the 3/8-inch-long soccer shoe[27] appeared to reduce the risk of injury.[28]

Catastrophic injuries are of great concern in football, and, since the 1976 rule changes prohibiting "spearing" (the use of the head and neck as the point of contact), they are now very infrequent (Table 21). Torg et al[29] reported a significant reduction in the frequency of fractures, dislocations, subluxations of the cervical spine, and quadriplegia in a recent 10-year period. The incidence of intracranial hemorrhage in their study appeared to increase, but this may be related to the availability of more sophisticated diagnostic techniques. The fatality rate from intracranial causes has not appeared to change. In 1984, for every 100,000 high school participants, the risk of cervical fracture, dislocation, or subluxation was 3.9, for quadriplegia .43, for intracranial hemorrhage 1.73, and for death from head and neck trauma .65. Mueller and Blyth[30] reported a significant overall reduction in fatalities in high school football. This was reflected by the 20 fatalities that occurred in 1965 compared to the four fatalities in 1985.

Permanent disability from catastrophic head and neck injuries are the most devastating injuries at higher levels of football competition, but chronic residua can result from less severe injuries. Semon and Spengler[31] demonstrated a rate of spondylolysis in college football players three times greater than the general population. Twenty-seven percent of the players with spondylolysis complained of chronic low back pain. Albright et al[32] found a 35% incidence of cervical spine abnormalities due to trauma on radiographic studies of college freshmen. Moretz et al[33] found that after 20 years, 39% of individuals who sustained knee injuries in high school persisted with significant knee symptoms, and 50% of this group had radiographic abnormalities. Those who did not sustain injuries were no more likely to have symptoms than individuals who did not play football. It appears that although football is a sport of great enjoyment and excitement, participation at higher levels of competition is associated with a significant acute injury rate and a real potential for permanent disability.

Basketball

Basketball is one of the more popular sports played in the United States both interscholastically and recreationally. There is little information regarding the injury experience of preadolescent players. Zaricznyj et al[6] reported that for school-aged children basketball was the fourth leading cause of injury in the nonorganized setting, behind football, rollerskating, and baseball, and the fourth most common cause of injury in community teen sports. In school-organized teams, the injury rate was 10.2%. This ranked basketball as the fourth leading cause of injury, behind football, wrestling, and gymnastics. The finger, ankle, and hand were most often injured.

At the high school level, more information about basketball is available, but it is still limited. Garrick and Requa[8] found a 31% injury rate in boys basketball (eighth highest sport) and a 25% injury rate in girls basketball (12th highest sport). Chandy and Grana,[10] using a more strict definition of injury, found a 6% injury rate in boys basketball and an 8% rate for girls. The ankle, knee, and leg were most often injured. Girls had a significantly higher incidence of knee injuries, and boys had a significantly greater chance of sustaining shoulder injuries. Moretz and Grana[34] found a high prevalence of ankle sprains in both male and female high school basketball players. They also found that females had a decidedly higher rate of total injury (76% to 16%) and of significant injury (18% to 8%). The greater susceptibility of females to injury in basketball has also been noted at the professional level,[35] and although the ankle sprain prevails as the most common injury, the female knee appears to be uniquely at risk. Gray et al,[36] in a case review study of female basketball players, found a five times greater frequency of anterior cruciate ligament ruptures in females than in males.

Wrestling

Wrestling is a sport that is extremely popular at the interscholastic high school level, ranking as the fourth or fifth most popular sport with several hundred thousand participants. The risk of injury in wrestling occurs as a result of the combative, collision components of the sport. As described by Snook,[37] injuries arise from direct blows from an opponent, from friction upon hitting the mat, from falls particularly during a takedown, and from twisting and leverage forces during controlling maneuvers.

Preadolescents and early adolescents have become active in wrestling, but there are few studies that have evaluated their injury experiences. Hartman[38] surveyed a group of preadolescent wrestlers and found only trivial injuries except for a metacarpal fracture. Strauss and Lanese[39] evaluated a group of 291 early adolescent wrestlers, with an average age of 12.3 years, and found an injury rate of 3.8 per 100 wrestlers and an average of two injuries per 100 matches. The torso was most often injured, followed by the upper and lower extremities. He found a significantly higher rate for high school (11%) and college (13% to 14%) wrestlers; these older competitors had more lower extremity and head and neck injuries. This study again emphasized that younger competitors have a different injury experience than those in higher levels of competition.

Requa and Garrick[40] studied 234 high school wrestlers who required even minimal care and determined an injury rate of 75%, second only to football. The rate of significant injury (15%) was similar to football. Sprains and strains were the most common injuries, with the site of injury well distributed between the upper extremity (29%), the lower extremity (33%), and the spine and trunk (34%). Spine strains and knee sprains were common, as were acromioclavicular sprains. In this study of all high school sports, only football had a higher incidence of injuries requiring surgical correction. Variables related to injury included previous injury, particularly to the shoulder, knee, and ankle, and being at the disadvantage during the takedown maneuver. Most injuries occurred during competition (43%) rather than in practice (37%) or scrimmages (20%).

Estwanik and Rovere[41] studied the 2-year experiences of 1,091 high school wrestlers in North Carolina. He found an overall injury rate of 23%. As in the previous study, the shoulders and knees were most susceptible to significant injury. Shoulder injuries, including acromioclavicular sprains and joint subluxations and dislocations, occurred most often while the wrestler was down on the mat and the arm used as a lever, or when the wrestler fell. Knee injuries, usually to the medial collateral ligament or the medial or lateral meniscus, resulted from forces delivered during the takedown or when in hyperflexion while on the mat. This study also demonstrated that the hand was susceptible to fractures and ulnar collateral ligament sprains, and the elbow to sprains and dislocations. "Cauliflower ears" were found to be decreasing in frequency because of head gear and improved mat surfaces, and severe neck strains and fractures appeared to be controlled by the strict rule against slams. Minor back and neck strains were a common injury, as were facial lacerations. No mention was made of skin infections from mat friction burns.

An additional source of injury to wrestlers is the strict calorie and fluid restriction employed to attain a weight felt to be most advantageous (see Chapter 10). The potential long-term impediments to normal growth and development and the detrimental acute effects on the response to exercise makes this a practice that requires careful monitoring and control.[42]

Soccer

Soccer has grown significantly in popularity in the United States in the last 2 decades, with approximately 1,600,000 children and adolescents participating in youth leagues and 220,000 in high school programs.[43] This growth has been greatest in the younger age groups, where the sport has been seen as an alternative to football in the fall, and baseball in the spring. Soccer is not classified as a collision sport, but most injuries arise from direct contact with a player, the ball, or the ground. Due to the running and kicking demands of soccer, overuse syndromes also are prevalent.

Studies of preadolescent and early adolescent soccer players indicate a low risk of injury. In a group of participants less than 12 years of age, Sullivan et al[44] found an injury rate of less than 1%. The lower extremity was most often injured, and contusions were the most common type of injury. McCarroll et al[45] found similar low rates of injury for 10 and under (1.9%), 12 and under (3.1%), and 14 and under (5.3%) participants. The ankle, knee, and shin were most often injured, and sprains and contusions were most prevalent. No mention was made in either study of epiphyseal fractures or injuries resulting in permanent disability.

For older adolescent participants, either in high school interscholastic programs or organized youth leagues, the risk of injury increases significantly. In the previously cited studies, injury rates increased to 7.7% for high school participants,[44] and to 6% for 16 and under, and 8.7% for 19 and under players in a community league.[45] Both studies demonstrated that the lower extremity, particularly the ankle, knee, and shin, was most often injured and accounted for over two thirds of the injuries. The remainder are evenly distributed between the upper extremity and the head and neck.

Significantly, the older competitors sustained more frequent severe injuries,[45] particularly injuries to the knee. Surgical intervention for medical collateral or anterior cruciate ligamentous sprains or for meniscal injury was not uncommon, and the risk for an injury to cause internal derangements of the knee appeared to occur about as frequently in soccer as in football.[46] Ankle injuries were usually sprains; shin injuries were usually contusions; and thigh injuries were most often strains or contusions.[47] Fractures most commonly occurred at the distal radius, and concussions, although uncommon, were reported. Adolescent females appeared to be at greater risk for injury than were adolescent males.[44,47] Goalkeepers had a higher than expected incidence of injuries, and midfielders a lower than expected rate.[44] Penalties and poor field conditions predisposed to injury.

Case reviews and general discussions have delineated specific problems unique to soccer. Smodlaka[48] discussed the potential danger of repeated heading of the soccer ball. The risk could not be quantified, but the potential for brain injury from the cumulative effect of repeated heading must be considered. The use of a lighter waterproof molded synthetic leather ball that is covered with urethane was suggested for children. Strong stabilizing neck muscles may reduce the force of impact. Burke et al[49] discussed eye injuries in soccer, most common in adolescent players. The most frequent injuries were hyphemas, vitreous hemorrhages, and corneal abrasions, and, although these injuries were not as severe as in racquetball or hockey, he suggested protective eye guards. Leach and Corbett[50] discussed three cases of anterior tibial compartment syndrome resulting from direct kicks and collisions, and emphasized the need for early diagnosis and treatment and protection of the lower leg. Smodlaka[51] reviewed the unusually high incidence of groin pain in soccer players. His review of case studies revealed the most common causes to include traumatic tendinitis or myositis of the adductor muscle, arthritis of the symphysis, and necrosis or osteitis of the pubis. Dental injuries also appeared to be increasing.

The popularity of soccer for children in the United States has been based, in part, on the hope that the risk of injury would be less than that occurring in football. As described, the risk of injury for the preadolescent and early adolescent is quite small, but for older competitors, soccer is a demanding sport and significant injuries, particularly to the knee, do occur. Children who continue to play highly competitive soccer well into adulthood have significantly increased the risk of developing chronic knee pain and radiographic evidence of osteoarthritis.[52]

Skiing

Each year approximately 5 to 12 million skiers[53] can be found on the ski slopes enjoying a sport that provides the thrill of speed and the demands of coordination and balance. A large percentage of these skiers are children, and they are exposed to a risk of serious injury due to the large forces of impact that the velocity of their motion can produce when they fall or collide with an object. Additionally, the presence of a ski, acting as a lever arm and rigidly attached to the foot, further increases the potential for augmentation of the impact forces.[54] This becomes of particular importance if the ski is fixed to the ground at the time of contact. Skiing injuries have changed in the last 30 years, mostly for the better, but the number of injuries to children appears to be increasing as more children participate in the sport.

Skiing injuries are usually expressed in units of 1,000 skier days or the total number of skiers on the slopes for a given day. Between 1900 and 1961 skiing injuries averaged 7.4 per 1,000 skier days, but by 1971 to 1972 a reduction to approximately three injuries per 1,000 skier days had been noted.[55] The decrease appears to be related to improvements in ski boots and bindings as well as to the improved supervision and grooming of the slopes and better instruction, but absolute documentation that these are the causative variables is not available. Studies have indicated that children incur 22% to 33% of the total injuries.[56,57] Children between 11 and 16 years appear to have the highest injury rates, and 10 and under the lowest.[56,58] Females have a higher rate of injury than males, and more injuries appear to occur to the less advanced young skiers.[54,58]

In the last 30 years, the frequency of specific skiing injuries has changed in children. The frequency of metatarsal fractures, foot and ankle sprains, and lateral malleolar fractures has decreased significantly due to the introduction of the higher rigid boot. Spiral oblique and transverse boot top fractures of the tibia and fibula are now more prevalent.[54] No significant change has occurred in knee or upper extremity injuries, but due to the reduction in foot and ankle injuries, the proportion of upper extremity and trunk injuries has increased.[53] Sprains consist of approximately 50% of the injuries, followed by contusions and fractures.[58] Most often injured are the thumb, particularly the medial collateral ligament; the lower leg, foot, and ankle; and the knee. Children appear to sustain the same number of head and trunk injuries as adults, but adults have a higher incidence of upper extremity injuries, except at the thumb, where the frequency is equal.[57] Children sustain three times the frequency of lower leg injuries, particularly tibial fractures,[57] and with increasing age approach the adult rate of knee injuries. Young children sustain less severe knee injuries; teen-agers sustain more severe knee sprains, usually to the medial collateral ligament, and these approach adult levels.[56] Knee injuries account for approximately 20% to 25% of all injuries, and one quarter are usually strains greater than grade one.[56,57]

There are specific injuries that are unique to skiing. Lacerations account for 8% to 15% of skiing injuries[53] and frequently can be quite severe. They usually result from being struck by the ski and may be reduced by the current use of ski brakes instead of straps. Fractures of the midshaft of the fibula appear to be increasing in frequency and may result from overuse injuries rather than macrotrauma.[59] The ulnar collateral ligament of the metacarpophalangeal joint of the thumb is often sprained while falling clutching the ski pole. Total separation of the ligament from the base of the first phalanx can result, and this injury requires surgical correction. Gripping the pole outside the strap may reduce the frequency of this injury.[60] At least 18 cases of severe cervical injuries were recorded between 1978 and 1983 in children 7 to 17 years of age, resulting from falls, collisions, and aerial accidents.[61] Deaths are recorded each year.

Many variables have been related to skiing injuries although absolute documentation is lacking. These include improper settings for bindings,[62] fatigue,[54] improper instruction,[58] late afternoon skiing,[54] recklessness,[56] poor lighting,[55] skill level,[54] ice or heavy wet snow,[55] large moguls, flat light, inadequate supervision on the slopes,[55] use of ski straps,[59] and the improper adjustment of bindings on rental skis.[63] The variables listed should be discussed with parents and children as they provide the source for practical suggestions that may prevent one of the serious injuries that can arise from skiing.

Track

Track is a sport that places great conditioning demands on participants. The risk of injury is almost entirely from repetitive microtrauma and acute strains. Much has been written about running injuries, due in part to the general interest in jogging, but definitive studies are still required to resolve many of the most important issues.

The acute and chronic injury experience of the preadolescent runner is currently poorly defined in the literature. A study of 48 track and field athletes between the ages of 10 and 15 years found an overall injury rate of approximately 50% per year with two thirds of the injuries representing overuse syndromes. The lower leg was most frequently injured, followed by the knee, ankle, and thigh.[64] A questionnaire survey of young distance runners revealed an 18% incidence of injury with shin splints, low back strains, and thigh strains the most frequent problems reported.[65] In a study of interscholastic high school athletes, males had an injury rate of 33% per year and females 35% per year.[66] In that study the lower leg again was most often injured, followed by the thigh, knee, and ankle. Chronic inflammations and acute strains were the most common injuries.[65] A study of 237 high school track athletes revealed one injury for every 5.8 males and every 7.5 females. Sprinting (46%), distance running, activities before and after practice, and pole vaulting were most often associated with injuries. Posterior tibial syndrome, ankle sprains, and patellar tendinitis were the most common injuries. Athletes with higher performance levels were likely to be injured.[67]

Concern has been expressed for the potential of chronic musculoskeletal problems that can result from strenuous long-term training. These considerations have been particularly addressed to the child who has not yet reached physical maturity. Repetitive microtrauma to the articular cartilage resulting in chronic joint changes,[68] epiphyseal stress fractures resulting in growth disturbance,[69] delayed skeletal and sexual maturity,[70] persistence in running despite the early warnings of pain,[71] early burn-out,[72] permanent muscle damage,[73] and inadequate thermoregulatory mechanisms[74] have all been raised as issues to discourage children from attempting extremes of endurance activities. These considerations represent reasonable concerns, but no direct studies are available to demonstrate the actual risk to long-term development and health. In a long-term follow-up of 498 collegiate cross-country runners, there was no increased incidence of osteoarthritis of the hips and knees.[75] At this time, there is no conclusive evidence that high levels of endurance running will be detrimental to the growth plates of the lower extremity.[76] The potential exists, however, and long-term studies are required.

Many attempts have been made to determine those variables that may predispose to overuse running injuries. Variables such as age, gender, years running, anatomic characteristics, body build, experience, speed, biomechanics, lack of stretching, terrain, and running shoes have all been suggested as significant variables but currently lack conclusive scientific proof.[77-79] Future studies may document the importance of these variables. Psychologic factors,[80] sudden changes in the intensity of training,[81] prior injury,[82] and the frequency and amount of running[83] have documentation as variables directly related to injury, but these studies were performed with adults.

Gymnastics

Since the early 1970s, the popularity of gymnastics has increased significantly, particularly among girls, with a total of approximately 600,000 children participating at the interscholastic or club level. Gymnastics is a demanding sport creating the potential for both macrotrauma from falls and microtrauma from repetitive floor exercises and the use of apparatus. Additionally, many female participants engage in poor nutritional practices to maintain a reduced weight that may be advantageous for competition.

In a study of high school injuries, gymnastics ranked fourth behind football, wrestling, and softball, with an injury rate of 56%.[9] Club gymnastic programs, which represent a broad age range, have demonstrated rates of injury of between 12%[84] and 22%.[85] The lower extremity was most often injured, but injuries to the head, spine, and upper extremities were also common.[86] Sprains, strains, contusions, and fractures were the most common injuries encountered. Approximately half the injuries were macrotraumatic and half represented overuse syndromes.[84] Floor exercises and tumbling accounted for the greatest number of injuries, followed by the balance beam, uneven parallel bars, and vault.[85]

Specific injuries are common to gymnastics. Spondylolysis in the lumbar region is four times more common in gymnasts than in the general population.[86] The handspring vault and the back handspring and back walkover appear to create the greatest lumbar hyperextension stress.[87] The use of the upper extremity for weight bearing has made fractures and dislocations of the elbow a frequent injury,[88] and stress reactions of the distal radial epiphysis a common injury.[89] Knee injuries are most commonly patellofemoral articulation inflammations, but 18% of the gymnastics injuries presenting for care at a sports medicine clinic were sprains and 14% meniscal tears. At that clinic, 11.5% of the knee injuries required surgical intervention.[90]

Specific variables have been related to gymnastic injuries. Upper extremity injuries appear to be more severe when thick mats are not employed.[88] Gymnasts with the greatest skill and performing the hardest maneuvers sustain the most severe injuries.[84] Spotters are frequently not present when injuries occur,[84,88] and injuries appear to increase significantly when participants practice more than 20 hours per week.[91]

The use of the trampoline and the minitrampoline, for both recreation and training, has been a part of gymnastic programs. The risk of catastrophic cervical injuries resulting in quadriplegia[92] fostered the recommendation that the trampoline be used only for athletes with high levels of skill while under close supervision. Further evaluation has revealed that this elite group is also at risk for catastrophic injury.[93] The American Academy of Pediatrics has recommended that trampolines should *not* be part of routine physical education classes, as a competitive sport, nor should they be used in home or recreational settings (Appendix 4).

A final problem encountered by gymnasts is the combination of high levels of physical training with an attempt to maintain a thin, angular appearance by caloric restriction. These activities have been demonstrated to cause disturbed growth, weight loss, anorexia, and amenorrhea.[69,94] The long-term consequences of these alterations to normal growth and development remain to be determined.

Ice Hockey

Ice hockey is a sport that demands speed, coordination, and the willingness to accept and deliver contact. The use of skates, sticks, and pucks while playing on ice with constant contact between players and rigid goal posts and boards makes the risk of injury an intrinsic part of hockey. This risk has not diminished the popularity of the sport; the American Hockey Association of the United States has estimated that there are 300,000 children between the ages of 6 and 16 years participating on 12,000 community teams in the United States.[95]

Studies evaluating the overall injury experience in youth hockey are currently limited. Sutherland,[96] in 1976, before face masks were mandatory, studied 706 boys between the ages of 5 and 14 and found an injury rate of 2.4%, or one injury per 100 hours of participation. This compared to a rate of 20% or one injury per 16 hours of participation for 207 high school hockey players. Head and neck injuries were most common for the preadolescent (59%) and high school (68%) players; the lower extremities accounted for approximately 25% of the injuries in both groups. Lacerations and contusions were the most common injuries encountered. Disruptive knee injuries, groin strains, tibial fractures, acromioclavicular sprains, and shoulder dislocations were injuries more characteristic of college and professional players.[97,98] Hockey ranked second as a sport associated with epiphyseal fractures.[99]

Park and Castaldi[100] determined that at the high school level, 48% of the injuries in hockey resulted from body contact, 17% from the puck, 12% from the stick, and 7% from falls. By position, 68% of the injuries occurred to forwards, 30% to defensemen, and 2% to goalies. Sutherland[96] found that approximately one third of the injuries occurred as a result of illegal maneuvers.

The high incidence of head and neck injuries has been of great concern. In youth hockey, Wilson et al[101] found that 7% of the participants had sustained facial injuries at some point in their careers and that 54% of the high school players had incurred this type of injury. These were most often lacerations and nasal fractures caused by the hockey stick. Maxillary, mandibular, and zygomatic fractures were more commonly seen at the college and professional levels. Dental injuries were also common with one in 10 youth and high school players having lost one tooth during their careers. These injuries were also most often caused by the hockey stick. Pashby[102] found that 8% of hockey injuries were to the eye, and 14% of these injuries caused legal blindness. Eye injuries included soft tissue injuries, hyphemas, corneal abrasions, orbital fractures, iris, lens, choroidal, and retinal damage, and traumatic glaucoma. The hockey stick again caused 74% of these injuries and 60% of the injuries that caused blindness. As a result of these authors' findings, the American and Canadian Amateur Hockey Associations mandated the use of facial protection in 1976. Children, high school players, and college players must now wear full face masks with mouth guards. Facial and eye injuries are only rarely seen now that this safety equipment has been mandated.[103]

The frequent occurrence of brain injuries including concussions and even death resulted in the requirement for helmets, although currently designed helmets may not afford optimal protection.[104] Tator and Edmonds[105] suggested that the provision of head and face protection may be a factor in a seeming increase in cervical spine injuries in hockey, presumably as a result of a change in the style of play. This association has yet to be proven. Quadriplegia, in their study of Ontario hockey players, had a frequency several times greater than that reported for football.

Prevention

The previous section has summarized the risk of injury in several sports. This information is essential in evaluating the medical needs of sports programs and helping parents and children select sports. Variables that are etiologically related to injury are essential to permit preventive intervention, but epidemiologic research is still required to clearly define causative factors. Several areas for injury prevention have been defined and should be considered when discussing sports participation (Table 22).

1. *Proper conditioning.* Appropriate conditioning of aerobic endurance, muscular strength, muscular endurance, flexibility, and the capacity to acclimate to heat prior to the competitive season should permit the athlete to better withstand the stresses of his or her sport. Preseason conditioning has been demonstrated to reduce the number and severity of knee injuries in football,[106] and carefully monitored warm-up, stretching, and cool-down has been shown to reduce the frequency of soccer injuries.[107]

2. *Avoidance of excesses in training.* Excessive training, sudden changes in training, or training for multiple sports at the same time can impose stresses that exceed the tolerance of the musculoskeletal system. Parents and athletes should be advised to avoid these practices, and they should be instructed not to ignore the early signs of pain. Excessive training has been documented to be a significant variable in the etiology of running injuries.[80,82]

3. *Appropriate competitive environment.* A safe well-maintained area for sports participation can reduce the risk of injury. Athletes participating on surfaces that are less than optimal can be injured by falls that otherwise would not occur. Ski slope grooming[54,55] and the condition of the snow[60] have been shown to be significant variables in skiing injuries, and the condition of the playing field has been demonstrated to be a factor in football injuries.[28]

4. *Resolution of a prior injury.* Athletes who have sustained an injury are more likely to be injured than athletes with no injury history. This has been demonstrated in football,[25] wrestling,[40] and track.[81] Variables such as psychologic traits, participation time, and morphologic charac-

teristics may be related to this association, but the incomplete resolution and rehabilitation of an injury may well be the most important causative factor. Athletes should be advised that before they return to competition, injured areas should be adequately healed and rehabilitated to the degree required to meet the demands of their specific sport. A physician's approval for a return to competition should be mandatory after a significant injury, and athletes who sustain permanent residua from an injury should be considered for protective bracing or redirection to another sport.

5. *Appropriate supervision.* Appropriate supervision of athletes, either by medical personnel, coaches, or supervisors, can reduce the risk of injury. These individuals can ensure correct training and conditioning techniques, provide prompt and effective medical treatment, and demand that only safe activities are permitted. Ski slope supervisors,[54,55] spotters in gymnastics,[84,88] and physicians and physiotherapists in soccer[108] are examples where close supervision of sports activities have reduced injury rates. The availability of certified trainers in high schools should also provide a mechanism to reduce injuries.

6. *Rule changes.* A careful evaluation of the causes of injuries in specific sports can permit the rules of the sport to be modified to eliminate unsafe practices. Disallowing slams in wrestling[41] and spearing in football[28-30] has had a significant effect in reducing severe neck injuries. Continued surveillance of individual sports should permit future modifications that may well reduce existing injury rates.

7. *Instruction in correct biomechanics.* The motions of sports place a repetitive stress on the musculoskeletal system. With correct biomechanics these stresses can be minimized as the body functions in a unified fashion. Incorrect biomechanics may place excessive stress on one specific area causing an eventual injury. An example is the higher incidence of elbow problems in pitchers with incorrect biomechanics.[109]

8. *Appropriate equipment.* Children who participate in sports should be made aware of the availability of safety equipment that can reduce the risk of injury. They should also be advised that this equipment should be in excellent condition and appropriately fit to their specific requirements and size. Equipment such as the headgear in wrestling, the face mask in hockey, the batting helmet and rubber spikes in baseball, and bindings and boots in skiing have all been effective in reducing injury rates. The removal of dangerous equipment, such as the trampoline, has also been effective in reducing injuries to the young athlete.

9. *Complete preparticipation physical assessment.* Prior to engaging in competitive athletics, children should receive a complete physical appraisal by a physician to determine if their selected sport is appropriate[110] (Chapter 4). During such an evaluation, medical problems that

may require exclusion from a sport or a modification of medical management can be evaluated. Residual musculoskeletal abnormalities from prior injuries can be assessed, and structural characteristics that may predispose to injury can be detected. Additionally, the child can be advised of any deficits in fitness parameters after body composition, muscular strength, muscular endurance, cardiovascular endurance, and flexibility are evaluated.

10. *Appropriate matching of competitors.* Children who participate in collision sports should be appropriately matched for fair and safe competition. This matching should take into consideration age, weight, and the stage of physical maturation. The latter is frequently overlooked, despite the well-established marked changes that occur in height and growth velocity, strength, body composition, and aerobic endurance that occur during the phases of adolescent sexual and physical development. The careful matching of competitors may represent an important variable for the low injury rates in youth football.[22]

REFERENCES

1. Clarke KS. Premises and pitfalls of athletic injury surveillance. *J Sports Med*. 1976;3:292-295
2. Caldwell F. Epidemiology takes its place on the sports medicine team. *Phys Sportsmed*. 1985;13:135-140
3. Walter SD, Sutton Jr, McIntosh JM, Connolly C. The etiology of sport injuries: a review of methodologies. *Sports Med*. 1985;2:47-58
4. Mendryk SW. A critique of accident and injury reporting methodology. *Can J Appl Sport Sci*. 1978;3:1-3
5. DeHaven KE. Athletic injuries in adolescents. *Pediatr Ann*. 1978; 7:704-714
6. Zaricznyj B, Shattuck LJ, Mast TA, Robertson RV, Delia G. Sports related injuries in school-aged children. *Am J Sports Med*. 1980;8:318-324
7. Gallagher S, Finison K, Guyer B, et al. The incidence of injuries among 87,000 Massachusetts children and adolescents: results of the 1980-81 statewide childhood injury prevention surveillance system. *Am J Pub Health*. 1984;74:1340-1347
8. Garrick JG, Requa RK. Injuries in high school sports. *Pediatrics*. 1978;61:465-469
9. Shively RA, Grana WA, Ellis D. High school sports injuries. *Phys Sportsmed*. 1981;9:46-50

10. Chandy TA, Grana WA. Secondary school athletic injury in boys and girls: a three-year comparison. *Phys Sportsmed*. 1985;13:106-111

11. Adams JE. Injury to the throwing arm: a study of traumatic changes in the elbow joint of boy baseball players. *California Med*. 1965;102:127-132

12. Gugenheim JJ, Stanley RF, Woods GW, Tullos HS. Little League survey: the Houston study. *Am J Sports Med*. 1976;4:189-200

13. Larson RL, Singer KM, Bergstrom R. Little League survey: the Eugene study. *Am J Sports Med*. 1976;4:201-209

14. Torg JS, Pollack H, Sweterlitsch P. The effect of competitive pitching on the shoulders and elbows of preadolescent baseball players. *Pediatrics*. 1972;49:267-272

15. Francis R, Bunch T, Chandler B. Little League elbow: a decade later. *Phys Sportsmed*. 1978;6:87-94

16. Grana WA, Raskin A. Pitcher's elbow in adolescents. *Am J Sports Med*. 1980;8:335-336

17. Barnes DA, Tullos HS. An analysis of 100 symptomatic baseball players. *Am J Sports Med*. 1978;6:62-67

18. Hale CJ. Protective equipment for baseball. *Phys Sportsmed*. 1979;7:59-63

19. Dickman GL, Hassan A, Luckstead EF. Ventricular fibrillation following baseball injury. *Phys Sportsmed*. 1978;6:85-86

20. Roser LA, Clawson DK. Football injuries in the very young athlete. *Clin Orthop*. 1970;69:219-223

21. Goldberg B, Rosenthal PP, Nicholas JA. Injuries in youth football. *Phys Sportsmed*. 1984;12:122-132

22. Goldberg B, Rosenthal PP, Robertson LS, Nicholas JA. Injuries in youth football. *Pediatrics*. 1988;81:255-261

23. Alles WF, Powell JW, Buckley W, et al. The National Athletic Injury/Illness Reporting System: 3-year findings of high school and college football injuries. *J Orthop Sports Phys Ther*. 1979; 1:103-108

24. Moretz A, Rashkin A, Grana WA. Oklahoma high school football injury study: a preliminary report. *J Okla State Med Assoc*. 1978;71:85-88

25. Blyth CS, Mueller FO. When and where players get hurt. *Phys Sportsmed*. 1974;2:45-52

26. National Athletic Trainers Association. *National high school injury registry*. Greenville, NC; 1986

27. Torg JS, Quedenfeld T. Effect of shoe type and cleat length on incidence and severity of knee injuries among high school football players. *Res Q*. 1971;42:203-211

28. Mueller FO, Blyth CS. North Carolina high school football injury study: equipment and prevention. *J Sports Med*. 1974;2:1-10

29. Torg JS, Vegso JJ, Sennett B, Das M. The National Football Head and Neck Injury Registry: 14-year report on cervical quadriplegia, 1971 through 1984. *JAMA*. 1985;254:3439-3443
30. Mueller FO, Blyth CS. An update on football deaths and catastrophic injuries. *Phys Sportsmed*. 1986;14:139-142
31. Semon RL, Spengler D. Significance of lumbar spondylolysis in college football players. *Spine*. 1981;6:172-174
32. Albright JP, Moses JM, Feldick HG, Dolan KD, Burmeister LF. Non-fatal cervical spine injuries in interscholastic football. *JAMA*. 1976;236:1243-1245
33. Moretz JA, Harlan SD, Goodrich J, Walters R. Long-term followup of knee injuries in high school football players. *Am J Sports Med*. 1984;12:298-300
34. Moretz A, Grana WA. High school basketball injuries. *Phys Sportsmed*. 1978;6:91-95
35. Zelisko JA, Noble HB, Porter M. A comparison of men's and women's professional basketball injuries. *Am J Sports Med*. 1982;10:297-299
36. Gray J, Taunton JE, McKenzie DC, Clement DB, McConkey JP, Davidson RG. A survey of injuries to the anterior cruciate ligament of the knee in female basketball players. *Int J Sports Med*. 1985;6:314-316
37. Snook GA. The injury problem in wrestling. *Am J Sports Med*. 1976;4:184-188
38. Hartmann PM. Injuries in preadolescent wrestlers. *Phys Sportsmed*. 1978;6:79-82
39. Strauss RH, Lanese RR. Injuries among wrestlers in school and college tournaments. *JAMA*. 1982;248:2016-2019
40. Requa R, Garrick JG. Injuries in interscholastic wrestling. *Phys Sportsmed*. 1981;9:44-51
41. Estwanik JJ, Rovere GD. Wrestling injuries in North Carolina high schools. *Phys Sportsmed*. 1983;11:100-108
42. American College of Sports Medicine. Position stand on weight loss in wrestlers. *Med Sci Sports*. 1976;8:xi-xiii
43. Keller CS, Noyes FR, Buncher CR. The medical aspects of soccer injury epidemiology. *Am J Sports Med*. 1987;15:230-237
44. Sullivan JA, Gross RH, Grana WA, Garcia-Moral CA. Evaluation of injuries in youth soccer. *Am J Sports Med*. 1980;8:325-327
45. McCarroll JR, Meaney C, Sieber JM. Profile of youth soccer injuries. *Phys Sportsmed*. 1984;12:113-117
46. Pritchett JW. Cost of high school soccer injuries. *Am J Sports Med*. 1981;9:64-66
47. Nilsson S, Roaas A. Soccer injuries in adolescents. *Am J Sports Med*. 1978;6:358-361

48. Smodlaka VN. Medical aspects of heading the ball in soccer. *Phys Sportsmed.* 1984;12:127-131
49. Burke MJ, Sanitato JJ, Vinger PF, Raymond LA, Kulwin DR. Soccerball-induced eye injuries. *JAMA.* 1983;249:2682-2685
50. Leach RE, Corbett M. Anterior tibial compartment syndrome in soccer players. *Am J Sports Med.* 1979;7:258-259
51. Smodlaka VN. Groin pain in soccer players. *Phys Sportsmed.* 1980;8:57-61
52. Chantraine A. Knee joint in soccer players: osteoarthritis and axis deviation. *Med Sci Sports Exerc.* 1985;17:434-439
53. Johnson RJ, Ettlinger CF, Campbell RJ, Pope MH. Trends in skiing injuries: analysis of a 6-year study (1972-1978). *Am J Sports Med.* 1980;8:106-113
54. Ellison AE. Skiing injuries. *Clin Symp.* 1977;29:1-40
55. Tapper EM, Moritz JR. Changing patterns in ski injuries. *Phys Sportsmed.* 1974;2:39-48
56. Blitzer CM, Johnson RJ, Ettlinger CF, Aggeborn K. Downhill skiing injuries in children. *Am J Sports Med.* 1984;12:142-147
57. Ungerholm S, Engkvist O, Gierup J, et al. Skiing injuries in children and adults: a comparison study from an 8-year period. *Int J Sports Med.* 1983;4:236-240
58. Garrick JG, Requa RK. Injury patterns in children and adolescent skiers. *Am J Sports Med.* 1979;7:245-248
59. Tapper EM. Ski injuries from 1939 to 1976: the Sun Valley experience. *Am J Sports Med.* 1978;6:114-121
60. Carr D, Johnson RJ, Pope MH. Upper extremity injuries in skiing. *Am J Sports Med.* 1981;9:378-383
61. Oh S. Cervical injury from skiing. *Int J Sports Med.* 1984;5:268-271
62. Ungerholm S, Gierup J, Gustavsson J, Lindsjo U. Skiing safety in children: adjustment and reliability of the bindings. *Int J Sports Med.* 1984;5:325-329
63. Ungerholm S, Gustavsson J. Skiing safety in children: a prospective study of downhill skiing injuries and their relation to the skier and his equipment. *Int J Sports Med.* 1985;6:353-358
64. Orvva S, Scarela J. Exertion injuries in young athletes. *Am J Sports Med.* 1978;6:68-72
65. Watson MD, Dimartino PP. Incidence of injuries in high school track and field athletes and its relation to performance ability. *Am J Sports Med.* 1987;15:251-254
66. Rowland TW, Walsh CA. Characteristics of child distance runners. *Phys Sportsmed.* 1985;13:45-53
67. Requa RK, Garrick JG. Injuries in interscholastic track and field. *Phys Sportsmed.* 1981;9:42-49

68. Micheli LJ, Micheli ER. Children's running: special risks? *Ann Sports Med.* 1985;2:61-63
69. Godshell RW, Hanson CA, Rising CA. Stress fractures through distal femoral epiphysis in athletes: a previously unreported entity. *Am J Sports Med.* 1981;9:114-116
70. Malina RM. Menarche in athletes: a synthesis and hypothesis. *Ann Hum Biol.* 1983;10:1-24
71. Green RG, Grange JJ. Drive theory of social facilitation: twelve years of theory and research. *Psychol Bull.* 1977;84:1267-1288
72. American Academy of Pediatrics, Committee on Sports Medicine. Risks in long distance running for children. *Phys Sportsmed.* 1982;10:82-86
73. Hagerman FC, Hikida RS, Staron RS, Sherman MS, Costill DL. Muscle damage in marathon runners. *Phys Sportsmed.* 1984;12:39-48
74. Bar-Or O. Climate and the exercising child: a review. *Int J Sports Med.* 1980;1:53-61
75. Sohn RS, Micheli LJ. The effect of running on the pathogenesis of osteoarthritis of the hips and knees. *Med Sci Sports Exerc.* 1984;16:150. Abstracted
76. Caine DJ, Linder KJ. Growth plate injury: a threat to young distance runners? *Phys Sportsmed.* 1984;12:118-124
77. Powell KE, Kohl HW, Casperson CJ, Blair SN. An epidemiological perspective on the causes of running injuries. *Phys Sportsmed.* 1986;14:100-114
78. Brody DM. Running injuries. *Clin Symp.* 1980;32:1-36
79. Warren BL, Jones CJ. Predicting plantar fasciitis in runners. *Med Sci Sports Exerc.* 1987;19:71-73
80. Crossman J. Psychosocial factors and athletic injury. *J Sports Med Phys Fitness.* 1985;25:151-154
81. Grana WA, Coniglione TC. Knee disorders in runners. *Phys Sportsmed.* 1985;13:127-133
82. Koplan JP, Powell KE, Sikes RK, Shirley RW, Campbell CC. An epidemiological study of the benefits and risks of running. *JAMA.* 1982;248:3118-3121
83. Pollock ML, Gettman LR, Milesis CA, Bah MD, Durstine L, Johnson RB. Effects of frequency and duration of training on attrition and incidence of injury. *Med Sci Sports.* 1977;9:31-36
84. Weiker GG. Injuries in club gymnastics. *Phys Sportsmed.* 1985; 13:63-66
85. Garrick JG, Requa RK. Epidemiology of women's gymnastics injuries. *Am J Sports Med.* 1980;8:261-264
86. Jackson DW, Wiltse LL, Cirincoine RJ. Spondylolysis in the female gymnast. *Clin Orthop.* 1976;117:68-73

87. Hall SJ. Mechanical contribution to lumbar stress injuries in female gymnasts. *Med Sci Sports Exerc.* 1986;18:599-602
88. Priest JD, Weise DJ. Elbow injury in women's gymnastics. *Am J Sports Med.* 1981;9:288-295
89. Roy S, Caine D, Singer KM. Stress changes in the distal radial epiphysis in young gymnasts: a report of twenty-one cases and a review of the literature. *Am J Sports Med.* 1985;13:301-308
90. Andrish JT. Knee injuries in gymnastics. *Clin Sports Med.* 1985; 4:111-121
91. Pettrone FA, Ricciardelli E. Gymnastic injuries: the Virginia experience 1982-1983. *Am J Sports Med.* 1987;15:59-62
92. Rapp GF, Nicely PG. Trampoline injuries. *Am J Sports Med.* 1978;6:269-271
93. Torg JS, Das M. Trampoline and minitrampoline injuries to the cervical spine. *Clin Sports Med.* 1985;4:45-60
94. Caine DJ, Lindner KJ. Overuse injuries of growing bones: the young female gymnast at risk? *Phys Sportsmed.* 1985;13:51-64
95. Sim FH, Simonet WT, Melton LJ, Lehn TA. Ice hockey injuries. *Am J Sports Med.* 1987;15:30-40
96. Sutherland GW. Fire on ice. *Am J Sports Med.* 1976;4:264-269
97. Hayes D. Hockey injuries: how, why, where and when. *Phys Sportsmed.* 1975;3:61-65
98. Feriencik K. Trends in ice hockey injuries: 1965 to 1977. *Phys Sportsmed.* 1979;7:81-84
99. Benton JW. Epiphyseal fracture in sports. *Phys Sportsmed.* 1982; 10:63-71
100. Park RD, Castaldi CR. Injuries in junior ice hockey. *Phys Sportsmed.* 1980;8:81-90
101. Wilson K, Cram B, Rontal E, Rontal M. Facial injuries in hockey players. *Minn Med.* 1977;60:13-19
102. Pashby TJ. Eye injuries in Canadian hockey: phase II. *Can Med Assoc J.* 1977;117:677-678
103. Pashby TJ. Eye injuries in Canadian amateur hockey. *Am J Sports Med.* 1979;7:254-257
104. Benoit BG, Russell NA, Richard MT, Hugenholtz H, Ventureyra EC, Choo SH. Epidural hematoma: report of seven cases with delayed evolution of symptoms. *Can J Neurol Sci.* 1982;9:321-324
105. Tator CH, Edmonds VE. National survey of spinal injuries in hockey players. *Can Med Assoc J.* 1984;130:875-880
106. Cahill BR, Griffith EH. Effect of preseason conditioning on the incidence and severity of high school football knee injuries. *Am J Sports Med.* 1978;6:180-184
107. Ekstrand J, Gillquist J, Moller M, Oberg B, Liljedahl SO. Incidence of soccer injuries and their relation to training and team success. *Am J Sports Med.* 1983;11:63-67

108. Ekstrand J, Gillquist J, Liljedahl SO. Prevention of soccer injuries: supervision by doctor and physiotherapist. *Am J Sports Med.* 1983;11:116-120
109. Albright JA, Jokl P, Shaw R, Albright JP. Clinical study of baseball pitchers: correlation of injury to the throwing arm with method of delivery. *Am J Sports Med.* 1978;6:15-21
110. Goldberg B, Saraniti A, Witman P, Gavin M, Nicholas JA. Preparticipation sports assessment: an objective evaluation. *Pediatrics.* 1980;66:736-745

Table 19. Injury Rates in Youth Sports for All Activities[5-8]

Age (years)	Rate (%)	Significant Injury (%)
6-12	3	20
13-19	7-11	20

Table 20. Highlights of Common Sports Injuries in Children and Adolescents

Baseball
1. Elbow and shoulder overuse injuries are the most frequent.
2. Chronic pathologic changes in the elbow and shoulder are very uncommon before adolescence.
3. Contact and collision injuries are infrequent.
4. Deaths have resulted from cardiac damage secondary to nonpenetrating chest trauma.

Football
1. At the youth level, significant injury occurs to 10% of participants. The hand or wrist and knee are the most common injury sites. Fractures and sprains are the most common types of injury, and surgery is rarely required.
2. At the high school level, significant injury occurs in 12% to 17% of participants. The knee and ankle are the most common injury sites. Sprains and strains are the most common types of injury, and surgery is required for 4% of players.

Basketball
1. The ankle is most commonly injured.
2. Female basketball players appear to be at greater risk of developing significant knee injuries.

Table 20. Highlights of Common Sports Injuries in Children and Adolescents *(continued)*

Wrestling
1. The preadolescent injury experience is different from that of older wrestlers.
2. High school wrestlers are most likely to sustain knee sprains, back strains, and shoulder injuries.
3. "Cauliflower ears" are decreasing in frequency.
4. Surgical correction is frequently required for injuries that are sustained.

Soccer
1. Youth soccer is associated with a low rate of injury (2%-5%).
2. Adolescent players have a higher rate of injury (6%-9%).
3. The ankle, knee, and forefoot are most often injured.
4. Significant knee sprains are not uncommon.
5. Repeated heading of the soccer ball may cause brain injury.

Skiing
1. Children incur 22%-23% of the total skiing injuries.
2. Metatarsal fractures, foot and ankle sprains, and lateral malleolar fractures have decreased in frequency.
3. Spiral and transverse boot top fractures are now more prevalent.
4. Significant knee injuries occur with increasing frequency as children get older.
5. Ulnar collateral ligament sprains of the thumb are common.

Gymnastics
1. Injury rates are between 12%-22%.
2. The lower extremity is most often injured.
3. Half the injuries are macrotraumatic and half are due to overuse syndromes.
4. Spondylolysis occurs four times more often than in the general population.

Hockey
1. Youth hockey injury rates are 2%-3%; high school rates are 25%.
2. Lacerations and contusions are the most common injury.
3. Facial injuries have been significantly reduced since the use of the face mask was mandated.
4. Cervical spine injuries may be increasing.

Table 21. Catastrophic Injuries in Football

Injury	Year		
	1976	1980	1984
Cervical spine fracture	110	62	42
Cervical quadriplegia	34	16	5
Intracranial hemorrhage	12	12	21
Craniocerebral fatality	12	11	9
Overall fatalities	28	13	9

Table 22. Factors to Be Considered in the Prevention of Injuries

1. Proper conditioning.
2. Avoidance of excesses in training.
3. Appropriate competitive environment.
4. Complete resolution of a prior injury.
5. Appropriate supervision.
6. Rule changes.
7. Instruction in correct biomechanics.
8. Appropriate equipment.
9. Complete preparticipation physical assessment.
10. Appropriate matching of competitors.

CHAPTER 12

OVERUSE SYNDROMES

Overuse syndromes[1,2] represent a broad spectrum of injuries caused by repetitive microtrauma to the musculoskeletal system from excessive or biomechanically incorrect activity. The anatomic structure sustaining the injury may be bone, tendon, ligament, bursae, fascia, muscle, or, uniquely in the child, growing cartilage. The latter can be either at a joint surface, at an apophyseal insertion of a muscular-tendon unit, or at the epiphyseal plate. The resultant types of injuries include stress fractures, tendinitis, fasciitis, sprains, bursitis, strains, and apophysitis. When recognized and treated promptly, these injuries can generally be expected to heal with no permanent residua. Chronic disability can potentially result when repetitive microtrauma persists, and this can result in growth deformity, osteochondritis dissecans, compartment syndromes, and chronic tendinitis or arthritis.

In past decades, overuse syndromes were problems unique to the older athlete, but with the explosion of sports participation by children, an increasing number of children are experiencing these injuries. It has been estimated that more than 20 million children are currently engaged in organized recreational activities, and many are engaged in high-level structured training programs. With young swimmers, runners, and other athletes practicing their sport for several hours each day, it is not unexpected to find overuse injuries increasing at a significant rate; in fact, they approach macrotraumatic contact injuries in frequency as the most common injuries sustained by young athletes. In a review of new injuries presenting at the Cleveland Clinic, Andrish[3] found that 40% of the new injuries in individuals less than 15 years of age were related to overuse of the involved area. Dominguez[4] found a 50% incidence of shoulder pain in young swimmers, and other researchers have found overuse syndromes to be common in sports such as baseball, track and field, gymnastics, and dance. With children's desire to participate, their dedication to excellence, and the push from parents and coaches, pediatricians should expect to see an increasing number of children with overuse injuries. To meet this medical need, the pediatrician must understand the causes of overuse syndromes, diagnose the type of injury, initiate appropriate treatment or make a suitable referral, and provide the young athlete with the information necessary to prevent potential or future problems.

Etiologies

The immediate cause of overuse syndromes is repetitive microtrauma to a specific anatomic site. There are several contributing factors (Table 23) that predispose a given child to develop this type of injury, and a careful history and physical examination will often explain the source of stress that created the cumulative microtrauma. Factors contributing to overuse syndromes follow.

1. *Modification of training techniques.* A significant change in a child's training routine may create pathologic stress. This may include a sudden increase in the intensity, duration, or frequency of training in an established sport; the addition of new conditioning programs, such as weight lifting; the simultaneous participation in a second sport; or recent heavy training in a newly selected sport, such as at a specialty camp.

2. *Incorrect biomechanics.* Many children never learn the correct biomechanics of a sport motion and, when they are required to perform their sport at a greater intensity, an overuse syndrome can result. This is frequently a factor, for example, in the shoulder problems of pitchers who lag their arm behind their bodies while throwing and in the leg pain of runners who have incorrect gait. Not uncommonly, a previously unresolved or unrehabilitated injury may force an athlete to modify otherwise correct biomechanics because of residual pain or muscle weakness.

3. *Improper environment.* Performing a sport on a surface that will not absorb and cushion impact is another factor in the development of overuse syndromes. This is most commonly seen in runners who repeatedly use hard inclined terrains; it also occurs in athletes in jumping sports, such as basketball or gymnastics, who leave the wood gymnasium floors to train outdoors on concrete surfaces.

4. *Anatomic malalignment.* Many children possess structural characteristics that are insignificant unless stressed by the demands of training for a specific sport. Leg length discrepancies of more than a 1/2 inch, femoral anteversion, valgus, varus or recurvation of the knee, increased Q angles, patella alta, bipartite patellas, excessive pronation, metatarsus adductus, cavus foot, and hallux valgus are examples of abnormalities of the lower extremity that can be factors in the development of overuse syndromes. A loose anterior capsule with a tight posterior capsule of the shoulder and tight lordotic backs[1] are other structural variants that can create abnormal stress from specific sport motions.

5. *Improper equipment.* Proper footwear is essential for the child who is engaged in a high-intensity running or jumping sport, and a failure to acquire optimal support, cushion, and stabilization can contribute to an overuse syndrome. The athletic shoe should have a high, firm heel counter, a pad for the Achilles tendon, flexibility in the forefoot, and adequate cushioning. A flared and beveled heel is important for runners.

The improper use of appropriate equipment, such as permitting shoes to wear significantly and using excessive resistance loads in strength training, can also create an overuse syndrome.

6. *Vulnerability of growth cartilage.* Children are unique in having growth cartilage at the epiphysis, the articular surface of joints, and the apophysis, the site of tendon-to-bone interface. Growth cartilage may be uniquely sensitive to stress.[2,5] This vulnerability can play a significant role in the development of such chronic sequelae of overuse injuries as bone deformity, microepiphyseal fracture, osteochondritis dissecans, and apophysitis. Individual children may be uniquely susceptible to apophysitis because of underlying cartilage dysplasia.[6]

7. *Growth.* Many overuse syndromes arise during adolescence; one factor predisposing teen-agers to overuse syndromes may be occurrence of a rapid growth spurt.[2] This sudden change in height will modify the relationship of the length of bone to the length of a musculotendinous unit. The resulting diminished flexibility can result in increased stress on the musculotendinous unit.

8. *Overtraining.* Overtraining,[7] an extreme of high-intensity training, has been recognized as a unique entity that results in wide fluctuations of body weight, insomnia, depression, anorexia, elevated resting heart rate, and delayed musculoskeletal recovery after exercise. The overtraining syndrome may be associated with an increased predilection for overuse injuries that compounds the factor of training intensity.

9. *Associated disease status.* Children with a medical problem that affects the musculoskeletal system may be predisposed to overuse syndromes.[1] These problems include, for example, tarsal coalition, spina bifida occulta, scoliosis, avascular necrosis, acquired arthritis, and intrinsic disease of muscle and collagen.

10. *Intrinsic vulnerability.* Many children participate at an intense level of physical activity and do not sustain an overuse injury, whereas others physically inactive and develop entities that are pathologically identical to overuse syndromes. This implies that other factors, such as cartilage-to-bone transformation, vascular integrity, specific tissue characteristics, or endocrinologic changes may play dominant roles in the development of an overuse syndrome in an individual child.

Principles of Treatment

Overuse syndromes represent a broad spectrum of injuries at different anatomic sites, but there are general therapeutic principles that are common to their management.[2,8] Initially, it would appear that repetitive stress creates an inflammatory reaction that evokes progressively increasing pain. With continued activity the inflammatory response proceeds to produce focal signs of swelling and tenderness. At this early inflammatory stage irreversible changes are unlikely if there is medical intervention. Continued activity can produce greater tissue damage and can result in the development of collagenous scars, enlarging epiphyseal microfractures, stress fractures, deterioration of articular cartilage, bony deformity, or avulsion of a musculotendinous unit. It becomes apparent that early medical intervention is the optimal management of overuse syndromes.

Treatment is initially directed at reducing the inflammatory response and permitting the injured area to heal primarily. The degree of tissue damage should determine whether complete rest or a modification of activity is indicated. Most athletes will comply best when some activity is permitted, and this should be specifically prescribed. An alternative choice includes a less intense training program that includes similar activities that will not stress the injured area. Examples include low-resistance biking with toe clips or running in water for lower extremity injuries. Activities that exercise noninjured sites, such as swimming, weight lifting, or rowing offer another alternative. The use of modified activity will prevent a degree of the deconditioning effects of complete rest although occasionally complete rest and immobilization are mandatory.

Reducing the inflammatory response can also be aided by physical therapy modalities and anti-inflammatory medications. There are a wide range of modalities that are designed to diminish swelling, pain, and muscle spasm and to increase blood flow. The superiority of one is yet to be established. Cryotherapy consists of noncompressed ice over the site for 30 to 40 minutes three times a day or 50° to 65° cold whirlpools twice daily. Therapeutic heat can also be efficacious, using either hot packs, whirlpool, or ultrasound. Contrast baths, alternating ice and heat in a two-to-one ratio, combines both modalities. Transcutaneous electric nerve stimulation appears to be effective in the relief of pain and spasm. The choice of a specific therapeutic modality is usually based on the clinical experience of the physician, physical therapist, or certified athletic trainer.

Anti-inflammatory medications have a role in overuse syndromes when they are dictated by symptoms of chronic pain and swelling and when the child is under the care and control of a physician who is monitoring the clinical course and the activity level. They should not be used to permit a child to return to activity without an appraisal of the degree of tissue damage. The medications include either an appropriate anti-inflammatory dosage of a salicylate or a nonsteroidal anti-inflammatory agent[9] (Table 24) used either continuously for several weeks or sporadically when the symptoms dictate. The choice of drug should be determined by the age of the child, the clinical response, the experience of the physician, and the risk of toxicity of the specific drug. When using a salicylate, the physician should always alert the athlete to discontinue the medication if any signs of influenza or varicella develop. The physician should not prescribe the drug during an influenza epidemic. Dimethyl sulfoxide (DMSO),[10] a topical anti-inflammatory agent, should not be employed for young athletes until its efficacy and safety have been established. The one-time use of inject-able steroids has a very limited role for children, and repeated injections are contraindicated.

When the injured area has healed, which usually requires 3 to 12 weeks, the athlete must be reconditioned before returning to full com-petition. This requires gradual cardiovascular and strength training, as well as a return of full flexibility, and performance skill must be pro-gressively reestablished. Most importantly, a review must be made of potential factors that predisposed to the overuse injury. Training tech-niques should be evaluated and biomechanical errors corrected. The training environment and the athletic equipment should be made opti-mal. An evaluation should be made for anatomic malalignment and, when possible, this should be corrected with conditioning, orthotics, heel lifts, or bracing. The child's muscle strength should be appropriate and balanced, and flexibility should be established in areas that are unusually tight, either because of recent rapid growth or intrinsic factors.

Common Overuse Syndromes

Apophysitis of the Posterior Calcaneus (Sever Disease)

Apophysitis of the posterior calcaneus, or Sever disease, is a chronic inflammation in the area of the insertion of the Achilles tendon.[11,12] Symptoms include pain around the heel, usually at the insertion of the Achilles tendon at the calcaneal apophysis or underneath the calcaneus. Symptoms are worsened during the heel strike of running. Radiologic studies may reveal fragmentation and sclerosis of the calcaneal apophysis although clinical symptoms often do not correlate with radiographic findings.

The etiology of Sever disease remains uncertain, but overuse appears to play a role. The landing foot for lay-ups in basketball or the stabilizing foot in soccer are often involved. Initial treatment consists of self-limited rest, ice, anti-inflammatory drugs, and a 1/4-inch cushioned heel lift for shock absorption and for limiting stress on the insertion of the Achilles tendon. Progressive stretching of the Achilles tendon should follow the initial therapy. Care should be taken in shoe selection to ensure proper fit of the heel counter, and old shoes that have the worn heel lower than the toe should be discarded.

Plantar Fasciitis

The plantar fascia, which runs from the calcaneus to the base of the proximal phalanges, can be strained, inflamed, or torn as a result of repeated stretching.[13,14] The symptoms of plantar fasciitis are often insidious in onset and consist of pain either in the arch or in the region of the heel where the medial head of the plantar fascia attaches to the calcaneus near the origin of the abductor hallucis. An Achilles tendinitis may also be present. The signs of plantar fasciitis include tenderness to deep palpation, most noted at the origin of the plantar fascia from the os calcis, particularly with the toes in dorsiflexion. Pain while toe walking is another frequent finding. Radiologic studies may reveal an associated, but clinically insignificant, traction spur from the lip of the calcaneus. The differential diagnosis includes a stress fracture of a metatarsal or the calcaneus, Sever disease, peroneus longus tendinitis, abductor hallucis myositis, rheumatoid disease, or entrapment of the posterior tibial or medial calcaneal nerve.

Plantar fasciitis can occur as a result of excessive running, running hills, speed work, biomechanical errors in the runner's gait, and the use of old, inadequate running shoes. Morphologic characteristics that include pes planus, cavus foot, excessive pronation, and a tight Achilles tendon may also predispose to plantar fasciitis. Treatment consists of altering the athlete's training to non-weight-bearing activities, rehabilitative modalities, arch support, anti-inflammatory medication, Achilles tendon stretching, and supportive taping of the arch. Particular attention should be directed to training techniques, the biomechanics of running, stretching, and shoe selection to prevent recurrence.

Achilles Tendinitis/Tenosynovitis

Achilles tendinitis[15,16] is an inflammation of the Achilles tendon that can be present at any point from the musculotendinous junction to the insertion on the posterior calcaneus. It usually results from repeated traction on the tendon, with the athlete progressing from pain after exercise to persistent discomfort throughout the day. The signs of Achilles tendinitis include local tenderness, usually at the malleolus level, crepitance while the foot is plantar flexed, and the presence of pain while toe walking and while the foot is plantar flexed against resistance. Although rare in children, a complete rupture of the tendon is represented by a gap in the tendon and a lack of any dorsiflexion of the foot upon squeezing the gastrocnemius muscle. Radiographic studies are usually negative except for a clinically insignificant traction spur at the posterior calcaneus. The differential diagnosis includes plantar fasciitis, Sever disease, plantaris rupture, peroneal tendinitis, stress fractures of the calcaneus, tibia, or fibula, and, most commonly, retrocalcaneal exostosis or bursitis (pump bumps).

Achilles tendinitis results from repetitive microtrauma from recurrent forceful traction. Predisposing factors that may be contributory include sudden intense training, excessive training, running with hard non-bending shoes, tight hamstring, soleus, and gastrocnemius muscles, weak anterior muscles of the forefoot, running on hard surfaces, and functional overpronation. Treatment consists of rest with an occasional need for brief periods of non-weight-bearing, rehabilitative modalities, anti-inflammatory drugs, and a firm 1/4-inch heel lift. This is followed by stretching, strengthening of the forefoot musculature, and a gradual return to activity. Orthotics may need to be prescribed. Prevention includes instruction in training techniques, the selection of cushioned shoes with properly fit heel counters, running on soft surfaces, changing direction when running on pitched surfaces, and proper stretching and conditioning.

Osgood-Schlatter Disease (Apophysitis of the Tibial Tubercle)

Osgood-Schlatter disease represents an apophysitis of the tibial tubercle, which may include a chronic patellar tendinitis at the insertion in the apophysis.[17,18] It is most common in boys where it occurs between the ages of 10 and 15 years; in girls it occurs between 8 and 13 years. Symptoms include pain over the tibial tubercle, which is usually exacerbated by activities that require repeated extension and flexion and by direct impact on the site. The child with Osgood-Schlatter disease exhibits tenderness and swelling over the tibial tubercle, and forced knee extension elicits pain. Radiographic studies reveal sclerosis, fragmentation, or separation with overlying soft-tissue swelling. Radiographic results frequently do not correlate with the clinical findings. The differential diagnosis includes bone tumor, cyst, pes anserinus bursitis, intrapatellar tendinitis, and a stress fracture of the proximal tibia.

The etiology of Osgood-Schlatter disease remains unclear, but sudden growth and the forceful traction pull of the extensor mechanism appear to play a role. Treatment usually consists of self-limited activity, ice, and protective knee pads. More aggressive therapy, including immobilization and surgical intervention, is rarely needed.[15] The disease is self-limited and ends when the proximal tibial epiphyseal plate closes. Stretching and strengthening of the quadriceps, heel cords, and hamstrings may be required if limitation of activity or immobilization has been required.

Shin Splints (Anterior Leg Pain Syndrome)

Anterior leg pain, or shin splints,[19,20] is a clinical syndrome represented by pain and discomfort between the tibial tubercle and ankle that results from repetitive running on hard surfaces or from forceful extensive use of the foot flexors. The source of pain may occur from an inflammation of the fibrous covering of bone, musculotendinous inflammation, or atypical stress fractures that are subroentgenographic. Symptoms consist of pain after activity that then progresses to persistent pain. The pain is usually linear and located along the anterior or posterior medial side of the distal one third of the tibia. Examination usually reveals local tenderness that is exacerbated by forced dorsiflexor contraction. Radiographic studies are usually unremarkable. Differential diagnosis includes a stress fracture of the tibia or fibula that may require a bone scan for definitive diagnosis. Most importantly, an anterior compartment syndrome either from trauma or overexertion must be considered. This is associated with diffuse pain and tenderness after exercise, a tense anterior compartment, anesthesia between the first and second toe, and a decrease in dorsiflexor strength. A failure to diagnose an anterior compartment syndrome can result in permanent muscle weakness and nerve damage.

The etiology of anterior leg pain appears to be a sudden increase in running for an inadequately conditioned athlete. Weak, inflexible anterior and posterior tibialis muscles, excessive pronation, poor biomechanics, and poorly fitting shoes have been identified as associated variables. Many modes of therapy have been employed to treat shin splints, but a cessation of running is the only consistently effective treatment. Alternative non-weight-bearing exercise can be employed during this period of rest. Heel pads, orthotics, stretching, anti-inflammatory drugs, casting, taping, strengthening the anterior and posterior tibialis muscles, and gait analysis may be helpful. Prevention of shin splints includes the avoidance of sudden increments in training, the avoidance of excessive hill work, the selection of proper stretching and strengthening programs, careful shoe selection, and correct coaching techniques in both biomechanics and conditioning.

Patellofemoral Syndrome ("Chondromalacia Patellae")

The patellofemoral syndrome,[21-24] sometimes called chondromalacia patellae, is a common disorder associated with anterior knee pain, which, in one third of the cases, is bilateral. Although often synonymous with chondromalacia, the latter implies true patellar articular cartilage pathology, represented by fibrillation, softening, and frank erosion. The symptoms of patellofemoral syndrome are anterior knee pain associated with exercise or afterwards, with prolonged sitting with the knees flexed, and with forced extension, squatting, or lifting; a feeling of grinding, locking, or giving way, and occasional swelling. The pain is usually localized to the anterior medial or lateral surface of the patella but may be described as being under the patella or actually inside the knee. Physical examination usually reveals a full range of motion of the knee but with pain elicited in full flexion. Tenderness on palpation of the margins of the patella and crepitation and pain while compressing the patella are frequently found. Radiographic studies include a posterior/anterior, lateral, and tangential view of the patella. The configuration of the patella and the sulcus angle should be radiographically evaluated, as should the relationship between the patella and the patella tendon. Radiographic studies exclude other pathologic states such as bone tumors. The differential diagnosis includes arthritis, discoid meniscus, suprapatellar plicae, osteochondritis dissecans of the medial femoral condyle, meniscal tears, infrapatella fat pad lesions, quadriceps or patella tendon tendinitis, infrapatellar tendon bursitis, recurrent patellar subluxation or dislocation, osteochondral fracture, peripatella soft-tissue inflammation, or bipartite patella.

The patellofemoral syndrome arises from excessive patellar compression. Although an acute traumatic episode may be the primary cause, it usually occurs insidiously from cumulative overuse. Many variables have been associated with patellofemoral syndrome, and these include training errors, inappropriate exercises, and improper biomechanics as well as anatomic characteristics that result in abnormal patellar tracking. The latter include an increased Q angle of greater than 20°. The Q angle is the angle formed from a line drawn from the middle of the patella to the center of the tibial tubercle and from the middle of the patella to the anterior superior iliac spine. Other anatomic characteristics include tibial torsion, pronation of the foot, abnormal patellar shape, abnormal sulcus angle, quadriceps weakness or contracture, particularly of the vastus medialis, patella alta, patellar instability, hamstring and heel cord tightness, and excessive internal hip rotation. Therapy is directed at reducing the inflammatory response and modifying the underlying anatomical pathology. Reducing the inflammatory response requires a reduction in activity, anti-inflammatory therapy, and physical therapy modalities, most often ice. When symptoms subside, an active exercise program to strengthen and stretch the hip and lower leg muscles should be pursued.

Strengthening generally begins with electric stimulation, when available, or with isometric exercises, and proceeds to an isokinetic program with apparatus such as an Orthotron or Cybex. If the latter are not available, a straight-leg-raising program, with weight suspended from the ankle, can be employed. The motions of hip abduction, adduction, extension, and flexion should be instituted first. When three sets of 15 repetitions with 10 pounds are attained, knee extension-flexion, limited to the final 30° to 40° of knee extension, can be added. This allows emphasis on the vastus medialis. Knee extension/flexion between 90° and 130° should be avoided until symptoms are fully resolved. Generally, free weights must exceed 15 pounds at 15 repetitions before a beneficial gain can be expected. Additional benefit can be gained by the use of orthotics, when excessive pronation exists, or patellar stabilizing braces such as the Palumbo or Marshall brace when anatomic abnormalities indicate their use. Surgical intervention may be required when conservative measures fail. Preventive measures include proper training techniques, correct biomechanics, avoidance of full squats and running stairs and hills, careful shoe selection, and careful strength and flexibility training. Preselection of athletes with anatomic risk for patellofemoral syndrome during a preparticipation evaluation can allow the institution of these preventive measures as well as permit the early prescription of ice, orthotics, and braces.

Shoulder Impingement Syndromes

Impingement of the shoulder[25-27] results from an inflammatory response created by the repeated stress of abducted, overhead motion, such as in throwing a ball or swimming. The rotator cuff musculature, particularly the supraspinatous muscle, the subacromial bursa, and, because of its position, the biceps tendon become impinged and inflamed under the arch created in the posterior two thirds by the acromion and in the anterior one third by the coracoacromial ligament. The impingement usually occurs in the anterior component of the arch, under the anterior acromion, the coracoacromial ligament, and the acromioclavicular joint. The symptoms of impingement are often insidious in onset but can progress to continuous shoulder pain throughout the day and night. The pain is usually exacerbated by movement of the arm above the horizontal plane of the shoulders. The signs of impingement include a painful break in motion of the arm in the horizontal plane during abduction (hesitation sign), tenderness on palpation over the top of the humerus during internal rotation, pain elicited by abduction in the frontoanterior plane, pain and weakness during abduction against manual resistance, and pain as the abducted arm is lowered from 120° to 70°. Pain and weakness is relieved after 5 mL of local anesthetic is injected into the subacromial bursa (impingement test). Radiographic examination is usually negative in children, but in more advanced degrees of impingement a loss of bone is seen in the acromion and the greater tuberosity. The differential diagnosis includes recurrent subluxation, rim tears of the anterior glenoid, acromioclavicular joint separation, meniscus damage, referred neck pathology, skeletal or lung tumors, arthritis, synovitis, developmental problems of the coracoid and acromium apophysis, and proximal humeral physeal stress injury.

The cause of impingement of the shoulder is generally repetitive overuse in throwing sports and swimming. Pitching for many years can lead to hypertrophy of the humeral head, which can predispose to impingement as can a tight posterior capsule associated with a loose anterior capsule.[2] Other factors causing impingement include poor pitching or swimming biomechanics, breathing to only one side while swimming, using swim paddles, and poor mechanics in the tennis serve. Treatment, as with other overuse syndromes, is directed toward reducing the inflammatory response. In children, according to Neer and Welsh's classification,[28] a stage 1 impingement, consisting of reversible edema and hemorrhage, is almost always the pathologic entity present. Stage 2 with thickening and fibrosis, and stage 3 with true tears, tendon rupture, and scarring are rare in childhood. A reduction of inflammation is accomplished by brief immobilization, physical therapy modalities, anti-inflammatory medication, prolonged modification of activity, and, for extreme situations, a one-time use of injectable steroids into a subacromial bursa. When symptoms have resolved, the shoulder should be rehabilitated with stretching of the posterior capsule and a strength program specifically directed at the rotator muscles, which are difficult to isolate unless specific positions are employed. A return to full activity should be gradual. Even with a stage 1 impingement, 6 months may be required for complete healing, rehabilitation, and a resolution of symptoms. When returning to activity any biomechanical or training errors should be corrected. Prevention consists of proper conditioning, correct biomechanical instruction, and the avoidance of excessive throwing during childhood. The early recognition of symptoms and the prompt institution of medical intervention may prevent a progression to irreversible changes and chronic residua.

"Little League Elbow" (Epiphysitis of the Medial Epicondyle)

"Little League elbow"[29-31] has traditionally been associated with an epiphysitis of the medial epicondyle caused by the repetitive strain of throwing. Associated findings may include aseptic necrosis of the radial head and capitellum, overgrowth of the radial head, and proximal radial epiphyseal closure. A strain of the flexor musculature and the pronator teres may also be present. The symptoms of "Little League elbow" consist of medial elbow pain that begins after throwing, but this can progress to be a chronic, persistent symptom. Examination reveals local tenderness over the medial epicondyle with possible extension to the flexor musculature. Wrist flexion against resistance may be painful, and full elbow extension may be limited. Radiographic studies may reveal fragmentation or separation of the medial epicondyle, trabecular and cortical thickening, overgrowth of the radial head, loose bodies, or osteochondritis dissecans. The differential diagnosis includes flexor or pronatore teres strain, Bennett fascial compression syndrome, ulnar collateral ligament sprain, and osteochondritis dissecans. The latter, a pathologic lesion of cartilage and bone that is most common on the anterolateral surface of the capitellum can result in loose body formation or arthritic changes.[32] This lesion may be a progression of the early stages of "Little League elbow." Older adolescent pitchers may develop true intra-articular pathology involving the radial capitellar joint or the trochlea.

Repetitive throwing creates a valgus strain at the elbow and requires a forceful flexion and pronation at the wrist. Improper warm-up, poor biomechanics, snapping curves and sliders, and excessive pitching are variables associated with the development of "Little League elbow." Treatment consists of rest followed by modified activity, physical therapy modalities, and anti-inflammatory drugs. Osteochondral lesions and frank avulsions may require surgery. When symptoms subside, stretching and strengthening of the musculature, particularly the wrist flexors, are indicated. Preventive intervention includes proper biomechanics, careful conditioning and warm-up, and a limitation on the amount of throwing. Early recognition and intervention is essential to prevent the progression to a chronic disability and intra-articular pathology.

Spondylolysis and Spondylolisthesis

Low back pain in the young athlete usually results from an acute traumatic event or from the chronic forces created by hyperextension, torsion, and compression. Athletes in sports such as football, weight lifting, gymnastics, wrestling, diving, and pole vaulting most often experience these symptoms. The pars interarticularis is frequently a site of repetitive microtrauma that can progress from a micro stress reaction to a true lytic lesion, called spondylolysis.[33-35] This defect, found in approximately 4% to 6% of the population with a definite genetic predisposition and three times more common in males than females, is found in the lower lumbar area. Symptoms consist of persistent and progressively worsening lower back pain, usually unilateral in location. Pain is exacerbated by motion, particularly twisting and hyperextension, and by vigorous physical activity. Physical examination may reveal paraspinous muscle spasm, localized pain, often described along the belt line, and an exacerbation of pain when the child is standing on one leg and hyperextending the back. Pain is usually alleviated by leaning forward, and nerve root irritation is not elicited by straight-leg raising. Radiographic studies may reveal a lytic lesion of the pars interarticularis (the "Scotty dog sign"), on an oblique view. Spina bifida in the fifth lumbar vertebra is often an associated finding. A technetium pyrophosphate radioisotopic bone scan may define the lesion. Treatment consists of a discontinuation of physical activity until pain subsides, usually taking between 6 weeks and 3 months. The use of a flexion antilordotic brace may hasten healing, and, when symptoms subside, abdominal muscle strengthening and lower body stretching should be recommended. The differential diagnosis includes a vertebral fracture, mechanical low back pain, a symptomatic lumbar disc, infection, Scheuermann disease extending distally to the second lumbar vertebra or lower, osteoid osteoma, osteoblastoma, or functional disease.

Spondylolysis may heal by bone union or by fibrous union and does not appear to predispose to back pain in later years of life. Occasionally, forward slippage of an upper vertebra on a lower vertebra can occur, creating spondylolisthesis. This lesion occurs more frequently in females than males and progresses most rapidly between the ages of 9 and 15, but can progress any time until vertical growth ceases. For this reason children with spondylolysis and, most importantly, spondylolisthesis, must be followed with serial lateral radiographs. Symptoms consist of persistent low back pain. Physical examination may reveal a variety of signs depending on the degree of slippage. These include paraspinous muscle spasm, tight hamstrings, inability to fully extend the hips, a short torso, heart-shaped buttocks, a low-appearing rib cage, and a high iliac crest. Radiographic studies can delineate the degree of slippage. Children with minor grade 1 slippage (of less than 25% forward displacement of one vertebra or another) should be placed on restricted activity until pain subsides, and they may benefit from a flexion antilordotic brace. After appropriate stretching and strengthening, they can return to all activities although frequently 6 months or more of rest may be required. If pain returns with a resumption of activity, the child should be referred to an orthopedic surgeon. When a slippage of up to 50% is present, children should be advised to avoid collision or contact activities that are associated with a potential for sustaining back injury. With this degree of slippage, fusion may have to be considered if symptoms of low back pain persist, and this must also be considered for any slippage of greater than 50%.[36]

REFERENCES

1. Harvey JS. Overuse syndromes in young athletes. *Pediatr Clin North Am.* 1982;29:1369-1381
2. Micheli LJ. Overuse injuries in children's sports: the growth factor. *Orthop Clin North Am.* 1983;14:337-360
3. Andrish JT. Overuse syndromes of the lower extremity in youth sports. In: Boileau RA, ed. *Advances in Pediatric Sport Sciences.* Champaign, IL: Human Kinetics Publishers; 1984:vol 1;189-202
4. Dominguez RH. Shoulder pain in swimmers. *Phys Sportsmed.* 1980;8:35-42
5. Bright RW, Burstein AH, Elmore SM. Epiphyseal plate cartilage: a biomechanical and histological analysis of failure modes. *J Bone Joint Surg.* 1974;56:688-703
6. Ippolito E. The osteochondroses: a new pathologic concept. *Ital J Orthop Traumatol.* 1984;10:203-216
7. Ryan J. Round table: overtraining in athletes. *Phys Sportsmed.* 1983;11:93-110
8. Stanish WD. Overuse injuries in athletes: a perspective. *Med Sci Sports Exerc.* 1984;16:1-7
9. Calabrese LH, Rooney TW. The use of nonsteroidal antiinflammatory drugs in sports. *Phys Sportsmed.* 1986;14:89-97
10. American Medical Association, Council on Scientific Affairs. Dimethyl sulfoxide: controversy and current status–1981. *JAMA.* 1982;248:1369-1371
11. Seder JI. Heel injuries incurred in running and jumping. *Phys Sportsmed.* 1976;4:70-73
12. Gregg JR, Das M. Foot and ankle problems in the preadolescent and adolescent athlete. *Clin Sports Med.* 1982;1:131-147
13. Furey JG. Plantar fasciitis: the painful heel syndrome. *J Bone Joint Surg (Am).* 1975;57:672-673
14. Roy S. How I manage plantar fasciitis. *Phys Sportsmed.* 1983;11:127-131
15. James SL, Bates BT, Osternig LR. Injuries to runners. *Am J Sports Med.* 1978;6:40-50
16. Clement DB, Taunton JE, Smart GW. Achilles tendinitis and peritendinitis: etiology and treatment. *Am J Sports Med.* 1984;12:179-184
17. D'Ambrosia RD, MacDonald GL. Pitfalls in the diagnosis of Osgood-Schlatter disease. *Clin Orthop.* 1975;110:206-209
18. Mital MA, Matza RA. Osgood-Schlatter disease: the painful puzzler. *Phys Sportsmed.* 1977;5:60-73
19. Andrish JT, Bergfeld JA, Walheim J. A prospective study on the management of shin splints. *J Bone Joint Surg.* 1974;56A:1697-1700

20. Jackson DW. Shinsplints: an update. *Phys Sportsmed.* 1978;6:50-64
21. Insall J, Falvo KA, Wise DW. Chondromalacia patellae: a prospective study. *J Bone Joint Surg.* 1976;58:1-8
22. James SL. Chondromalacia of the patella in the adolescent. In: Kennedy JC, Larson RL, eds. *The Injured Adolescent Knee.* Baltimore, MD: Williams and Wilkins Co; 1979:205-251
23. Dehaven KE, Dolan WA, Mayer PJ. Chondromalacia patellae in athletes. Clinical presentation and conservative management. *Am J Sports Med.* 1979;7:5-11
24. Malek MM, Mangine RE. Patellofemoral pain syndromes: a comprehensive and conservative approach. *J Orthop Sports Phys Ther.* 1981;2:108-116
25. Neer CS II. Impingement lesions. *Clin Orthop.* 1983;173:70-77
26. Brunet ME, Haddad RJ, Porche EB. Rotator cuff impingement syndrome in sports. *Phys Sportsmed.* 1982;10:86-94
27. McMaster WC. Painful shoulder in swimmers: a diagnostic challenge. *Phys Sportsmed.* 1986;14:108-122
28. Neer CS II, Welsh RP. The shoulder in sports. *Orthop Clin North Am.* 1977;8:583-591
29. Tullos HS, King JW. Lesions of the pitching arm in adolescents. *JAMA.* 1972;220:264-271
30. Pappas AM. Elbow problems associated with baseball during childhood and adolescence. *Clin Orthop.* 1982;164:30-41
31. Jobe FW, Nuber G. Throwing injuries of the elbow. *Clin Sports Med.* 1986;5:621-636
32. Pappas AM. Osteochondrosis dissecans. *Clin Orthop.* 1981;158:59-69
33. Wiltse LL, Widell EH, Jackson DW. Fatigue fracture: the basic lesion in isthmic spondylolisthesis. *J Bone Joint Surg.* 1975;57:17-22
34. Jackson DW. Low back pain in young athletes: evaluation of stress reaction and discogenic problems. *Am J Sports Med.* 1979;7:364-466
35. Ciullo JV, Jackson DW. Pars interarticularis stress reaction, spondylolysis and spondylolisthesis in gymnasts. *Clin Sports Med.* 1985;4:95-110
36. Wiltse LL, Jackson DW. Treatment of spondylolisthesis and spondylolysis in children. *Clin Orthop.* 1976;117:92-100

Table 23. Causes of Overuse Syndromes

1. Modification of training techniques
2. Incorrect biomechanics
3. Improper environment
4. Anatomic malalignment
5. Improper equipment
6. Vulnerability of growth cartilage
7. Growth
8. Overtraining
9. Associated disease states
10. Intrinsic vulnerability

Table 24. Dosage of Nonsteroidal Anti-inflammatory Drugs for Adolescents

Drug	Dosage (mg)	Frequency (times per day)	Mean Half-life (hr)
Ibuprofen (Motrin, Rufen)	600	4	2
Indomethacin (Indocin)	50	2-3	2-3
Naproxen (Naprosyn, Anaprox)	500	2	12-15
Piroxicam (Feldene)	20	1	38
Sulindac (Clinoril)	200	2	16-20
Tolmatin sodium (Tolectin)	400	4	1
DiClofenac sodium (Voltaren)	75	2	2

CHAPTER 13

THE TEAM PHYSICIAN

The team physician is an important part of any good athletic program. This discussion concerns itself mainly with high school programs, although it certainly applies to college programs as well. During the last 10 to 15 years, coaches and athletic directors have come to realize that good sports medicine care can improve team performance and make things easier for coaches. Ideally, the team physician is an integral part of the athletic program and should be involved in all aspects of it.

How does one become a team physician? In the past, physicians became involved because their children played on the team, and they gradually drifted into a relationship with the team and the coaches, but seldom pursued the development of a good sports medicine program. Today some team physicians are much more likely to be involved in a more formalized program and have specific responsibilities.

Necessary Components of an Athletic Medicine Program

Facilities

A good high school program needs to have a place where athletes can be diagnosed and treated. It should be separate from the locker room and have adequate space for several people. It should contain basic equipment such as a whirlpool, cold-packing material, examination tables, cabinets for equipment, and a sink. Good diagnosis and proper treatment cannot take place in a crowded locker room full of exuberant young athletes; therefore, it is important that the facility be separate, properly equipped, and able to be closed off.

Personnel

A critical part of a good athletic medicine program is a certified athletic trainer. The team physician should make a concerted effort to encourage the leaders of the program to obtain the services of a certified trainer. This is not always possible but it is not so far-fetched as it may seem. Across the country more and more states are mandating the presence of an athletic trainer in schools involved in interscholastic programs. A capable athletic trainer can make the job of the team physician much more pleasant by serving as the initial contact with the injured athlete and by conducting the rehabilitation program. The responsibility for the return-to-action decision must be borne by the team physician. However, the trainer will certainly play a strong role in this decision. During practice times, most team physicians are not available due to office commitments. This is where athletic trainers are invaluable: they treat injuries and are in close contact with the athletes. Proper communication between trainer and the team physician is essential. The physician needs to be kept up-to-date on athlete injury status so that decisions can be made as to treatment. The team physician must learn to depend on the trainer's ability, and together they form a "medical team."

Duties of the Team Physician

A formal written agreement and a job description are of value because they identify the physician as the person ultimately responsible for the athletes' medical care. The services may be rendered for pay or gratis, but a written agreement and a job description are very important. This can be accomplished with the athletic director, the school board personnel committee, the principal, or any official with the authority to create such documents. The document should clearly state that the physician has control over the acute care of the injured athletes, especially with regard to removal from competition and returning to play. This will reduce misunderstandings, and it actually should help the coach deal with athletes and/or parents upset about the necessity of keeping the athlete out of competition. It is unlikely that a school district would pay for the malpractice insurance coverage of a volunteer team physician, but, if the physician is not being reimbursed for rendering treatment at a game or practice, many states' "Good Samaritan Acts" specifically protect the volunteer team physician from liability.

Preparticipation Evaluation

The physician should be certain that every athlete has had proper evaluation. See Chapter 4 for a detailed discussion of the preparticipation evaluation. This is a good way to identify previous injuries that were not properly rehabilitated. Practically speaking, if there is not an athletic trainer available, a school nurse or other qualified medical person certainly should review the interval history forms (see Chapter 4) and be sure that the physician remains informed about previously injured athletes.

Establishment of Policy

There should be a document or policy statement outlining the entire athletic medicine program. This will ensure continuity of philosophy of care for the athletes, regardless of who is running the program. Appendix 5 is a self-appraisal checklist for school athletic programs that can be used as a guide for establishing such a policy.

Attendance at Team Activities

It would be helpful to have the team physician meet with the coaching staff before the season. Ideally, the physician would meet with the team before the season to discuss how injuries will be managed and to counsel about sport-specific health-associated hazards such as "making weight" by wrestlers and taking anabolic steroids by football players. In schools where the coaching staff meets with parents of the athletes, the physician could be part of this meeting also. This would enable parents to get to know the physician and develop confidence in the care that their young athletes receive.

It is impractical for most physicians to attend every practice, although such attendance could be helpful. A team physician should be present at all games involving contact collision sports since these are the high-risk sports (eg, football, ice hockey, wrestling, and possibly gymnastics). During a game, the team physician's authority must be absolute regarding treatment of injuries and return to play. This allows the coach to concentrate on coaching, without having to bear the responsibility for diagnosis and treatment of injured athletes.

At games, the physician should coordinate the activities of the sports medicine team, which may include rescue personnel, one or more trainers, student trainers, and the like. When a severe injury occurs, it is advisable to allow rescue personnel to provide immediate treatment and transport of severely injured athletes without interference. For example, a player who is down and complaining of neck pain may have sustained a cervical spine injury and should be moved only by trained rescue personnel, placed on a backboard, and transported properly. It is essential to have rescue personnel available to handle emergencies in the collision sports. If they are not physically present, the team physician must know the phone number of the emergency medical service and must know where the nearest available telephone is located.

A useful team physician's bag is a large tackle box, and a suggested list of equipment to be included is in Table 25. Other recommended equipment that should be available on site at collision sports events is listed in Table 26.

Who Can Be a Team Physician?

Physicians may feel that they must possess the skills of an orthopedic surgeon in order to be a team physician. This is not the case at all; primary care physicians with an interest in sports and young people can become very capable team physicians. Qualifications that may be helpful in obtaining this goal follow.

The team physician needs to have knowledge of the appropriate care of acute soft tissue injuries and be able to recognize and treat potentially serious injuries quickly and competently. Team physicians also should have knowledge of the sport they are covering because this has a direct bearing on the type of trauma that the young athlete may sustain. An understanding of nutrition for athletes is important in order to counsel the players about unwise practices such as eating steaks before an athletic event.

One should plan to attend continuing medical education courses on sports medicine whenever possible. Several journals are available providing information about various sports medicine topics. These are listed in the Suggested Reading list at the end of the chapter.

Physicians can learn a great deal about sports medicine from the athletic trainer if one is available in the school or college. Today's certified athletic trainers are college graduates with between 800 and 1800 hours of trainers' room time during their preparation. They have been rigorously screened and usually have very sound practical knowledge.

Medical Coverage of Athletic Events

Personnel

High-risk sports. A health professional should be in charge of medical activities at these athletic events. This person should be a health professional with an interest in the care of athletes who is, at a minimum, CPR certified and experienced in the management of acute trauma. An athletic team should have available the most qualified person willing to serve in this capacity. Such individuals include physicians, certified athletic trainers, EMTs, paramedics, and nurses.

Low-risk sports. A designated individual or coach who is certified for CPR and first aid should be in attendance at low-risk events.

Practices. At least one coach who attends all practices should be certified for CPR and first aid.

Emergency Plan

Ideally, a written emergency plan should be developed prior to the onset of the competitive season.

1. *Personnel.* If an emergency arises, it must be decided ahead of time who on the playing field will be responsible for assisting the insured athlete and who will be responsible for calling for help.
2. *Ambulance service.* The location of the closest emergency service and the closest hospital to the playing area must be determined.
3. *Activating the system.* The phone number and method of activating the emergency system should be discussed with all coaches and other personnel. The location of the nearest phone must be determined and, if it is a pay phone, coins should be attached to the written emergency plan. The plan and coins should be in a conspicuous place in the first-aid kit.

Event Coverage

1. Personnel available to provide medical coverage may vary from community to community. It is not always practical or necessary to have an emergency team and ambulance available, even for all high-risk sports events. Coverage will vary depending on the availability and expertise of the health providers in a community.
2. *Determining priorities.* When considering coverage, the two most important factors are (1) size of the audience (unless there are other plans for care of the spectators), and (2) the risk of serious injury to a participant.
3. *Injury risk.* Risk of injury to the participant can be based on available epidemiologic data (see Chapter 11). For example, the sports that need medical coverage most are the contact/collision sports (see Chapter 4) such as football, ice hockey, and wrestling; gymnastics, which is not a contact/collision sport, is associated with enough injuries that it also should be covered by an appropriate health professional.

SUGGESTED READING

Booher JM, Thibodeau GA. *Athletic Injury Assessment.* 2nd ed. St. Louis, MO: Mosby-Year Book, Inc; 1985

Clinics in Sports Medicine. Philadelphia, PA: WB Saunders Co. Periodical

Medicine and Science in Sports and Exercise. Baltimore, MD: American College of Sports Medicine. Monthly scientific journal

Physician and Sportsmedicine. Minneapolis, MN: McGraw Hill Publishers. Monthly peer-reviewed journal directed towards primary care physicians.

Shangold M, Mirkin G. *The Complete Sports Medicine Book for Women.* New York, NY: Fireside Books, Simon & Schuster, Inc; 1985

Smith NJ, ed. *Common Problems in Pediatric Sports Medicine.* Chicago, IL: Year Book Medical Publishers; 1989

Sullivan JA, Grana WA, eds. *The Pediatric Athlete.* Park Ridge, IL: American Academy of Orthopaedic Surgeons; 1990

Vinger PF, Hoerner EF, eds. *Sports Injuries.* 2nd ed. St. Louis, MO: Mosby-Year Book, Inc; 1986

Yearbook of Sports Medicine. Chicago, IL: Year Book Medical Publishers. Serial publication

Table 25. Contents of the Team Physician's Medical Bag

Pen light

Otoscope

Ophthalmoscope

Blood pressure cuff

Stethoscope

Gauze pads (2″ × 2″, 4″ × 4″)

Eye wash (sterile saline)

Adhesive tape – the most convenient is the 2″ width, although some should be 3″

Disposable plastic sandwich bags ("Baggies") for ice application

Elastic bandages – 2″, 4″, 6″

Arm/shoulder slings

Plaster of paris strips to make splints

Money for phone call

Aqueous epinephrine 1/1000

Albuterol inhaler for asthmatics

Acetaminophen

Tuberculin syringes and needles for injection of adrenalin if necessary

Tracheostomy equipment: 14-gauge angiocatheter or thyrotomy kit with cricothyroid cannula

Antibiotic eye ointment

A system for recording injuries – could be index cards or a notebook, each athlete having an individual page

Surgical closure-strips

Antibacterial solution for cleaning abrasions and lacerations

Eye patch for corneal abrasions

Prescription pad

Pens

Tongue blades

Tincture of benzoin in single-use vials to increase adhesiveness of tape

Oral airways (2 sizes)

Aluminum-foam splint for fingers

Bandage scissors

Bandaids

Rubber gloves to wear when in contact with blood

Table 26. Other Equipment Recommended for Collision Sports

Oxygen – portable, with valve, mask, and tubing
Ambu bag with mask
Cervical collar, stiff
Splints
Bolt cutter (for removal of football face mask)
Crutches
Spinal board with cervical immobilizer straps (if no emergency medical technician service in the community)

CHAPTER 14

REHABILITATION

Rehabilitation of a sports-related injury involves the principles of rehabilitating the injured part to maximum and safe function in the shortest time. In addition, three other principles are important in the rehabilitation of a sports-active person:

1. Deconditioning of the athlete should be minimized.
2. The opportunity for sport skill maintenance should be maximized.
3. Psychologic support should be provided.

Although most primary care physicians will not be supervising their patients' rehabilitative programs, they should be aware of the principles involved in rehabilitating athletic injuries.

The average soft-tissue injury that prevents athletes from participating in their sport may result in a significant loss of general cardiovascular and neuromuscular conditioning as well as depreciation of sports-specific skills. If a comprehensive approach is not planned, reconditioning and maximization of skills may require additional time after rehabilitation of the injured part prior to being ready to participate at the preinjury level.

The generally available therapeutic exercise equipment and physical modalities provide the physician/trainer/therapist the opportunity to direct the athlete for maximum cardiopulmonary conditioning, flexibility, general muscle strength, and endurance while rehabilitating the injured area. For example, if an athlete has sustained a knee injury and a period of immobilization and/or limited activity is required, it is possible to maintain cardiopulmonary, upper extremity, and contralateral leg conditioning with prescribed exercises and the use of various therapeutic exercise equipment. If the athlete is a figure skater and has sustained an upper extremity or shoulder girdle area injury, that person can return to skating at a lower level of complexity and intensity as soon as pain control is achieved. This maintains lower extremity strength and general conditioning. It may be a number of days or weeks before the individual is able to return to competitive skating. However, when the injured area is ready, the remainder of the athlete will be ready to resume a near preinjury level of participation.

The injured athlete must perceive a sense of continuing involvement in the sport as well as with teammates and coaches. If this is not sensed, the injured athlete usually feels rejected and may withdraw from team participation. He or she will be less enthusiastic about the total rehabilitation program and subsequent return to the sport. The injured athlete may remain a part of the team/sport environment as a scorekeeper, manager, or coaching assistant. The individual's involvement in the sport and the support and encouragement of colleagues are critical parts of the overall rehabilitation program.

Injury and Inflammation

An important concept in sports injury rehabilitation is that the effect of injury or inflammation is not limited to the local area of involvement. Injury and/or inflammation can cause a sequence of biologic events including pain, disuse, atrophy, and fibrosis. The potential consequences of these factors must be recognized in the planned rehabilitation program. If not, recovery will be delayed, performance compromised, and the probability of a recurring and more significant injury increased. One should consider these apparent individual concerns as part of a related continuum (Fig. 28).

Whenever there is inflammation or injury there is a period of pain and inhibitory disuse of the injured and adjacent areas. Whether caused by an external force or internal focal inflammation, the response is local pain and disuse. Continued pain and disuse result in clinical evidence of progressive weakness and atrophy. The biologic response of repair to noninfectious inflammation is fibroplasia. Fibroplasia will result in fibrosis and a lack of flexibility, in addition to a lack of strength. If these consequences are not treated, contracture may develop. The resultant limited excursion and existing weakness may cause altered function, usually a compensatory functional change observed as altered skill mechanics. Obviously, these changes have a deleterious effect on the quality of performance. One should not treat tendinitis with rest and anti-inflammatory medications and expect a complete recovery. Nor is it reasonable to treat the sprained medial collateral ligament of the knee by rest or immobilization and apply a brace for external support, and expect the athlete to return to competition. The principles of a sound rehabilitation program must apply to all aspects of the aforementioned cycle. The carefully planned rehabilitation program is responsive and attentive to all aspects of care, from acute injury to complete return to sports participation.

Guidelines for Sports Rehabilitation

It is helpful to divide the rehabilitation of a sports-related injury into five phases. These phases are independent of the consideration for minimizing deconditioning, maximizing skills, and providing psychologic support. They refer to rehabilitation of the injured and

adjacent anatomic areas. The five phases are
1. Acute injury
2. Initial rehabilitation
3. Progressive rehabilitation
4. Integrated functions
5. Return to sport

Before initiating a comprehensive rehabilitation program, it is important for the trainer/therapist to carefully review the history of the injury, the initial physical findings, and any changes that have occurred before assumption of care. Also, a review of anatomy and function of the injured area provides a framework for the phases of rehabilitation.

The physician treating athletes should know some of the common definitions of injury, sprains, and strains that ultimately influence the rate of progress during rehabilitation. Sprains are injuries to ligaments and fibrous capsular tissue, and strains are injuries to muscles, frequently musculotendinous junctions. The severity of sprains and strains is reported as Grades I, II, and III. However, there is a continuum from 0% to near 100% and, therefore, the subjective interpretation between grades will be variable from one examiner to another (Table 27). In addition to the subjective interpretation by the examiner, one must also correlate the injury with the pain tolerance of the injured individual, which contributes another significant variable to the evaluation process.

A common athletic injury is the sprained ankle, an inversion injury. The sprained ankle will be used as an example to discuss the guidelines for rehabilitation. The details of the mechanism of injury as well as the history of previous ankle injuries should be elicited prior to initiating treatment for the current injury. In addition to considering the two most frequently injured ligaments, the anterior fibulotalar and the fibulocalcaneal, the other anatomic areas of possible associated injury include the anterior ankle capsule, the peroneal retinaculum, tendon sheath and tendons, the physis of the distal fibula in a growing child, and the articular cartilaginous aspects of the fibulotalar joint. In a Grade I ankle sprain the damage is usually limited to the anterior fibulotalar ligament. In a Grade II ankle sprain it is likely that both ligaments are involved, although not equally, and there is probably additional injury in some of the other noted anatomic areas. In a Grade III ankle sprain there is probably significant injury to both anterior fibulotalar and fibulocalcaneal ligaments, as well as injuries to other soft tissues and probable articular cartilage compression. The extent of injury contributes to defining the range of time anticipated to achieve each of the phases of athletic injury rehabilitation (Table 28).

Phase I: Acute Injury

The goal of this phase is to stabilize the injured area, limit pain, and avoid additional injury. The treatment for acute soft-tissue injury is discussed in Chapter 16. The rationale for rest, ice, compression, and elevation (RICE) must be supplemented by support (S), a posterior splint of plaster or fiberglass or a commercially made ankle immobilizer. Immediately after injury, it may be difficult to differentiate between Grades I and II. Therefore, we strongly encourage some form of rigid external support to limit motion and avoid additional soft-tissue swelling, as well as to maintain the injured part in a comfortable position. Too often when a patient is evaluated for an ankle injury and the radiographs are negative for a fracture, the individual is advised that it is only a sprain. The ankle is wrapped with an elastic supportive bandage, and the patient is instructed to put an ice bag over the ankle every 3 or 4 hours. If this proves to be a Grade I or lesser injury, the treatment will have proven to be reasonable. However, if this proves to be a Grade II injury, the patient will probably experience unnecessary discomfort, additional swelling, and prolonged disability. In an obvious Grade III sprain, a posterior splint or commercially prepared immobilizer for support, protection, and immobilization should be considered mandatory. Local anesthetics should not be injected into injured areas for relief of pain. Instead, appropriate analgesics should be provided as indicated by the examiner's assessment of the extent of injury. The acute injury phase will last from 24 to 96 hours and is dependent on the location and extent of the injury.

Phase II: Initial Rehabilitation

The goal of this phase is to ensure the progressive, pain-free recovery of a maximum range of motion of the injured area. This is generally associated with a gradual decrease in the swelling. The pathologic process of early healing is associated with minimal tensile strength. Active-assisted complete range-of-motion (ROM) exercises should be instituted, but at the point of pain or discomfort, the range should be limited. As one approaches the end of Phase II, sufficient healing will have occurred to initiate limited-resistance, short-arc-range exercises.

It is generally recommended that the exercise treatment be preceded by 10 to 15 minutes of either cryotherapy or a warm pack, the choice determined by the extent and location of the injury and the preference of the therapist. Active-assisted ROM implies appropriate manual guidance by the examiner, as determined by the comfort of the individual and the response and sensitivity of the injured area. Early muscle recovery is encouraged by isometric exercises, a contraction without change in length, eg, quadriceps tightening and straight-leg raising.

The isometric exercises recommended for an ankle injury are directed to motions and muscles of eversion (peroneals), plantar flexion (gastrocsoleus), and dorsiflexion (anterior tibial). If one of the muscles is minimally responsive or nonresponsive, electric stimulation may be beneficial. Once the muscle is contracting well, electric stimulation is of minimal benefit. As progress is achieved toward the completion of the ROM, it is appropriate to initiate limited range, lightweight resistance exercise.

Phase III: Progressive Rehabilitation

The goals of this phase are to maintain a full ROM, increase strength of the injured area, and initiate limited-activity coordinated skills with appropriate protection. During this phase, there is a rapid change in the healing response and an increase in the tensile strength to approximately 50% of normal. At this time, it is appropriate to initiate isotonic progressive resistance exercises. Isotonic exercise represents a change in length of the muscle through part or all of its range against an existing force. These exercises are especially effective when the resistance is progressively increased. The concept of progressive resistance exercises generally consists of three sets of repetitions, with each repetition being held at its maximum point of excursion for five seconds. The initial resistance is submaximal, increasing to a near maximal load on the second set and to a maximal load on the third set. The rate of progression is determined by observing the response of the injured area and the individual's body language of discomfort. When the individual is able to complete three progressive sets of 15 repetitions without evidence of undue pain or abnormal biomechanics, it is time to gradually increase the resistance force. The muscle groups identified in Phase II are further strengthened in this phase. In addition, the other injured soft tissues are gradually stressed during the increased motion and resistance program.

In general, rehabilitation on specialized equipment is not recommended in the early stages of progressive resistance exercises. The use of assigned free weights limits the possibility of overexertion and reinjury. If unobserved, a competitive individual may seek the unwise additional weight resistance challenge in exercise equipment. A reinjury at this time will not only delay the overall recovery process but may cause additional injury and prolong the program. Therefore, careful guidance is indicated. When it is evident that the injured area is able to tolerate the increased resistance of free weights, the moderate use of exercise equipment is appropriate.

Near the end of the progressive rehabilitation stage, other modalities of strengthening, isotonic and/or isokinetic, are incorporated to permit a greater range of freedom and physiologic response in the exercise program. There is sufficient muscle strength, when compared with the noninjured side, to permit individual progression to simple coordinated skill exercises. For example, the program may include simple walking, jogging, and slow side steps. This progression provides the initial interaction of the injured area with other muscle groups, as well as the stimulation of the proprioceptive response to complex motions. This is the time to determine whether specific protection will be necessary to allow the individual's return to more comprehensive function. If needed, the specific supplemental external protection, eg, taping or braces, must be selected.

Phase IV: Integrated Functions

The goals of this phase are to maintain flexibility, increase strength, and increase and enhance the coordinated functional performance skills. Tissue healing has progressed to near 90% tensile strength, and proprioceptive responsiveness is being integrated with the coordinated activities of skill movement. The individual is jogging, starting simple crossover maneuvers, starting and stopping, using a tilt board, and progressing to sharp cuts and changes of direction at maximum speed. The coach becomes an important contributor to rehabilitation during this stage, as care begins to be transferred from a health professional to the coach. Thus, interaction between both professionals is critical.

Phase V: Return to Sport

During this phase, the major goal is to determine readiness for advanced skills and participation in the selected sport. The clinical sense of readiness for competition is subjective. Thus, the experience of the participant and the physician, trainer, and coach is necessary. The achievement of normal muscle strength is objective, either by hand test or recorded isokinetic test. It is imperative that the rehabilitation program continue until the person is advised to stop these specific exercises on a routine basis. In many instances, an injured area will require a continued program for as long as the individual plans to remain sports active and achieve maximum performance. It is important for the athlete to understand the rationale for the prolonged prescribed exercises to maximize his/her abilities. It is not necessary to have expensive exercise equipment to achieve an excellent result. The most elaborate exercise equipment does not simulate the forces and the activity of normal athletic participation. During this phase, the medical staff progressively transfers responsibilities for the athlete's performance to the coaching staff. The health professional's major role is to determine the continuing maintenance program that will maximize recovery and minimize the possibility of reinjury.

SUGGESTED READING

American Academy of Orthopedic Surgeons. *Athletic Training and Sports Medicine*. Chicago: American Academy of Orthopedic Surgeons; 1984

Arnheim DD. *Modern Principles of Athletic Training*. 6th ed. St. Louis, MO: Mosby; 1984

Basmajian JV, ed. *Therapeutic Exercise*. 4th ed. Baltimore, MD: Williams and Wilkins; 1984

Southmayd W, Hoffman M. *Sports Health*. New York, NY: Quick Fox; 1981

Table 27. Sprains and Strains Guidelines*

GRADE	I	II	III
Percent injury	0 – – – – – – – – –	25 – – – – – – –	50 – – – – – – –
Description	mild stretch	moderate partial tear pull	severe torn rupture
Observation Palpation	minimal swelling mild point tenderness no palpable defect	moderate swelling localized pain palpable abnormality defect	moderate to major swelling pain on limited examination palable defect
Stability	stable with minimal pain	instability with stress	instability during examination
Active motion	full with mild discomfort	pain with incomplete motion	pain with minimal motion
Functional activity	limited with discomfort	pain with attempt	incapable of
Associated injury	unlikely	probable at mild to moderate degrees	probable at severe degree multiple structures

*Pain tolerance is major unknown variable.

Table 28. Guidelines for Athletic Injury Rehabilitation*

Phase	Functional Goals	Pathologic Process	Rehabilitation Treatment	Responsible Person	Grade	Time (Days)
I: Acute injury	Protection limit injury limit swelling limit pain	Tissue injury Hematoma/tissue edema Inflammation	Rest Ice Compression Elevation Support	Health professional 100%	I II III	1-2 1-4 2-4
II: Initial rehabilitation	Complete pain-free ROM	Inflammation Early fibrosis Minimal tensile strength 0%-15%	Active-assisted ROM Limited short-arc resistance	Health professional 100%	I II III	1-4 4-10 7-10
III: Progressive rehabilitation	Maintain ROM Increase strength Limited activity skills Determine need for protection	Fibrosis Primitive collagen Increase tensile strength 15%-50%	Active ROM Flexibility Resistance Progressive resistance exercises	Health professional 100%	I II III	1-4 4-10 7-20

Phase	Goals	Tissue status	Interventions	Supervision	Grade	Time (Days)
IV: Integrated functions	Increase and enhance skill performance Increase strength Maintain flexibility	Maturing collagen tissue characteristics evident Tensile strength 50%-90%	Advance progressive resistance exercises Enhance flexibility Progress coordinated functions	Health professional 50% Coach 50%	I II III	1-4 4-10 7-14
V: Return to sport	Determine readiness for advanced skills and participation Simulated participation Prevent reinjury	Tissue-specific remodeling Tensile strength 90%-99%	Maintain strength and flexibility Progress coordinated motions Monitor protection	Health professional 25% Coach 75%	I II III	1-4 4-10 7-20

Total Grade	Time (Days)
I	5-18
II	17-44
III	30-78

*Other considerations: (1) other tissue injury; (2) pain tolerance; and (3) compliance

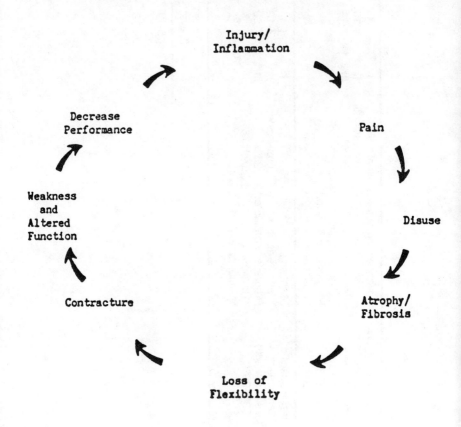

FIG. 28. Inflammation/Pain/Performance Cycle.

CHAPTER 15

THE ATHLETIC TRAINER

Historically, athletic trainers have been caring for competitors since the days of the early Greek Olympians. They were there to care for bruised and sore muscles, to rub and oil "their charge" before competition and bathe him afterwards, and to bandage and care for his injuries. The "rubber" was still part of the athletic scene in the first half of the present century. Many of these athletic trainers were individuals whose active athletic careers ended because of accident or age, or they had earned their way from locker room boy to equipment man to trainer. Many became proficient in mastering and developing athletic training techniques. Through reading, on-the-job training, and association with team physicians and other medical professionals, they created the foundations of the present-day professionally prepared, certified athletic trainer. Certification now is available through examination by the Board of Certification of the National Athletic Trainers Association, Inc.

Today athletic trainers are, through both college programs and clinical experience, well-prepared professionals in the following areas of health supervision: first aid and emergency care, injury recognition, treatment modalities and reconditioning, selection and fitting of protective equipment, nutritional needs of the athlete, athletic taping and wrapping procedures, the construction of special protective devices, athletic facility design and safety, use of medical records, and administration of athletic medical facilities. Some athletic trainers have advanced degrees in fields such as physical medicine and rehabilitation, and many have developed special areas of expertise (eg, biomechanical analysis, exercise physiology, muscle testing and performance evaluation, education, and research) within the area of sports medicine. Athletic trainers are required to accumulate Continuing Education Units by attending symposia, workshops, and lectures to update and enhance their skills. They work in a wide range of facilities and at various levels of medical care, including hospitals, sports medicine clinics, rehabilitation centers, and physicians' offices. Athletic trainers are employed in high school and college athletic programs, as well as with professional athletic teams and private athletic clubs.

In many athletic programs, the athletic trainer is administratively responsible for the overall operation of the sports medicine services. The trainer is on site on a daily basis and works in concert with the team physician, school physician, family physician, consulting physician, or other medical and paramedical professionals involved with the health care of the patient athlete.

The athletic trainer has become a respected professional in a health care delivery system for organized athletes. The major facet in this professional growth and competence has been the efforts of the National Athletic Trainers Association, Inc., to develop guidelines for the education and certification of athletic trainers. As a result of this growth, the medical boards of 20 states regulate the profession through licensure, registration, or certification (Table 29). In addition, four states regulate athletic trainers by exempting them from the Physical Therapy Practice Act (Table 30). Although it may present a formidable economic challenge for some schools, optimal care of the high school athlete requires the presence of a certified athletic trainer on staff. Moreover, he/she should be in attendance at practices and contests, especially the high-risk events such as football and wrestling.

Functions of the Athletic Trainer

The athletic trainer interacts with school administrators, coaches, equipment staff and other support staff, physicians (team, family, consultant), school nurses, paramedical professionals, teachers, parents, and the athletes themselves. The primary responsibilities of the athletic trainer are in the following four areas: (1) injury prevention, (2) first aid and emergency care, (3) treatment and rehabilitation, and (4) program administration.

Injury Prevention

Athletic trainers can be involved in the various screening and testing programs conducted before and during the season and can assist with the preparticipation medical evaluation (see Chapter 4). They can record height and weight, determine lean body mass (skin-fat folds), perform vision screening, determine blood pressures and pulse rates, and perform a musculoskeletal assessment including the degree of joint mobility or instability from a previous injury and the degree of functional impairment. Programs for weight control, nutrition counseling, heat acclimatization, and fluid balance can also be provided by the certified athletic trainer.

Protective taping, wrapping, and padding techniques are a traditional function of the athletic trainer. These procedures provide a means of protecting anatomic areas that are at risk because of previous injury, protecting recent injuries, and helping reduce the risk of injury.

The athletic trainer participates in selection and modification of protective athletic equipment and constructs special protective pads or devices to meet specific needs. He or she collaborates with the coaching staff in establishing conditioning programs during the preseason, inseason, and offseason times.

The athletic trainer can be responsible for surveying athletic sites to assess the safety of the area. Too often, athletes are disabled by avoidable accidents caused by chuckholes or rocks in the field, a bleacher that is too close to the out-of-bounds line, rigid yard markers too close to the sidelines, a broken bottle, an unpadded post at the end of a playing area, or even a slippery locker room or shower floor.

First Aid and Emergency Care

The best time to examine an athletic injury is immediately after it occurs, before excessive bleeding or swelling occurs, before protective spasm or pain develop, and before the body part is splinted by this protective pain and spasm.

The team physician may not be present during practices when most injuries occur. The athletic trainer may be the only person available to assess the nature and severity of the injury during this "golden period." The trainer is able to take an appropriate history of the injury and may even have witnessed the event. This information is an invaluable aid to the physician in establishing a diagnosis.

The athletic trainer is prepared to provide such first aid and emergency care as stabilizing an injured part (extremities or head and neck), providing care for abrasions and lacerations, and securing the appropriate emergency transportation. When necessary, the trainer can apply temporary tape sutures to a laceration until a physician can provide definitive care. Athletic trainers can provide immediate care for varying degrees of contusion, sprain, and strain. They have been trained to triage injuries, render the appropriate first aid or emergency measures, and render decisions regarding the level of emergency.

Treatment and Rehabilitation

Rehabilitation starts with the prevention of morbidity through quick and effective first aid measures. The control and prevention of hemorrhage, effusion, edema, inflammatory response, and spasm reduce the morbidity of the tissue at the injury site and facilitate the earliest possible return to full and safe participation.

The athletic trainer is skilled in using various physical modalities to reduce discomfort and facilitate a prompt reconditioning program. In consultation with the attending physician he or she will select the appropriate treatment modality and will initiate a planned program of reconditioning exercises to retain or restore range of motion, strength, power, endurance, and functional capability.

Because of the athletic trainers' thorough understanding of the special needs of the athlete, they can develop programs to meet the unique needs and demands of the athlete, which are usually far greater than those of the nonathlete with a similar injury. Trainers will individualize the care to meet the needs of athletes in each sport because each activity has its own special physical requirements and each individual his or her own special needs.

Program Administration and Implementation

Ultimately, the responsibility for what happens or fails to happen in a school sports medicine program rests with the team or school physician. The athletic trainer assumes directive responsibility from the team or school physician and administrators for the routine administration of the health care program and the prevention and treatment of injury to the players. When additional consultation or treatment is indicated he will assume the responsibility of assuring appointments in conjunction with the team physician and maintaining appropriate and accurate records.

Whenever an individual assumes such a critical role in an organization everyone must recognize the authority that is empowered to that individual, and that individual and others must be knowledgeable about the responsibility as well as the liability being assumed. The athletic trainer respects and welcomes the supervision and cooperation of his team physician and will maintain an open channel of information relating to the health care and status of all players. The relationship becomes one of mutual trust, respect, and confidence based on the recognition of the special contributions each can make to the program.

Athletic trainers have the first level of responsibility for medical care and were acting as physician-extenders or physician assistants long before the term was coined. They still assume this role within the limits of their competence and the confidence of their physician associates. Trainers can administer programs developed in cooperation with physicians in the following areas: record keeping; requisition and inventory of equipment and supplies; and liaison with coaches, administrators, and parents. They can organize the preparticipation physical examinations, develop communication and transportation programs for injury situations in contests and practice sessions, and train and supervise student aides. They can collect and analyze data on the incidence and severity of injuries by sport or by athlete, and assess causative factors and preventive measures.

The athletic trainer can be an associate to the physician; an ally to the coach; a peer to the administrator; a protector, friend, and confidant to the player; and a source of comfort to the parent, who has a continual concern about "who is taking care of my child."

Table 29. States Regulating Athletic Training (1990)

Delaware
Georgia
Idaho
Illinois
Kentucky
Louisiana
Massachusetts
Mississippi
Nebraska
New Jersey
New Mexico
North Dakota
Ohio
Oklahoma
Pennsylvania
Rhode Island
South Carolina
South Dakota
Tennessee
Texas

Table 30. States That Regulate Athletic Trainers by Exempting Them From the Physical Therapy Practice Act

Arizona
Connecticut
Hawaii
New Hampshire

CHAPTER 16

INITIAL MANAGEMENT OF MINOR SOFT-TISSUE TRAUMA*

The presentation of minor soft-tissue trauma in pediatric practice is a frequent occurrence. The patient is usually a child or youth who has received a blow to a muscle or bone during a game or practice resulting in a painful, swollen area (a contusion), or who may have "pulled" a muscle (a strain), or twisted a joint and injured a ligament (a sprain). Initial management of these minor injuries is fairly consistent regardless of whether it is a contusion, sprain, or strain.

Strains and sprains have been classified into three grades (Table 31, Fig. 29), and primary care physicians should be able to diagnose and treat all contusions and strains and at least the Grade I degree of sprain.

Rest, ice, compression, and elevation (RICE) are the classic components in the initial management of acute soft-tissue injuries. The athlete should be asked to return to the office for a reevaluation in two or three days if there has been little improvement with the following treatment.

Rest

Resting the injured area (and not the entire athlete) is quite important for the first 24 to 72 hours as movement can encourage further bleeding into the tissue. Unfortunately, athletes are quite likely to ignore the advice to rest. Frequently, the most successful way to rest a painful sprained ankle or contusion of the quadriceps muscle (a "charley horse") is to insist that the adolescent use crutches to avoid weight bearing. Resting a sprained ankle has been simplified by the development of inflatable splints, such as the Aircast® (Fig. 30), that prevent ankle eversion and inversion and can be removed for cryotherapy, sleep, and rehabilitative exercises that reduce swelling, improve range of motion, and prevent disuse atrophy of the muscles.

After 3 days, if there is residual pain, swelling, or tenderness, the physician should prescribe rehabilitative exercises because prolonged immobilization will produce disuse atrophy and consequent weakness of the muscle units helping to stabilize the joint, thus setting the stage for a reinjury. Most primary care physicians are unfamiliar with rehabilitative methods, but there is an abundance of medical literature on the subject.[1] Enlisting the aid of a certified athletic trainer, physiotherapist, or orthopedic surgeon may be necessary for optimal rehabilitation.

Ice (Cryotherapy)

The application of ice to injured tissues has been known since Hippocrates' time as being an effective way to decrease swelling and produce numbness. It has been used since at least the 18th century to produce enough local anesthesia to allow surgery such as lithotomy and amputation.

But does it work to treat acute injuries and inflammation? One of the few randomized studies of the effectiveness of cryotherapy used patients with acute ankle sprains that were severe enough to prevent them from bearing weight.[2] These subjects were randomized to receive either (1) cryotherapy beginning immediately; (2) cryotherapy beginning after 36 hours; or (3) heat treatments beginning immediately. Full activity was reached in 13 days, 30 days, and 33 days, respectively. This showed that not only was cryotherapy more effective than heat therapy, but that it needs to be applied as soon as possible after the injury.

We now understand cryotherapy's presumed mechanism of action on pain, muscle spasm, and edema. When the tissue temperature surrounding the site of the injury is decreased after the application of cold, nerve impulses and conduction velocity are diminished, with resulting diminution of pain. Muscle spasm of the surrounding area is diminished as muscle-spindle firing is suppressed. Its effect on edema is multifactorial. It is known that microhemorrhage frequently continues for several days after even minor tissue injuries, and the vasoconstriction induced by cryotherapy reduces blood flow into the area and decreases capillary permeability, thus limiting further hemorrhage. Subcutaneous and intramuscular hemorrhage can produce a secondary edema as the blood cells disintegrate, resulting in a disruption of local circulation with a consequent decrease in the supply of oxygen to the tissue. The oxygen demand of the cells can be diminished by decreasing their metabolism using cold, thus preventing further tissue death with resulting cell breakdown and further edema. However, continuing cryotherapy beyond 30 minutes can cause a reflex vasodilatation.

Chipped ice has been shown to be the most effective source of cold, a fortunate finding as it is also the cheapest and is usually readily available. The ice can be contained in disposable plastic sandwich bags. Flexible-gel cold packs are also useful and are somewhat easier to apply, but may not be as effective as ice.

The cold packs should be applied intermittently for the first 48 hours at least and should be applied for 20 minutes at a time, at least 3 to 4 times a day. An effective way to affix the ice pack is with an elastic bandage, but a single layer of wet bandage should first be applied to the skin to conduct cold while preventing frostbite and also to maintain some degree of compression (Fig. 31). The rest of the bandage is then used to hold the ice in place. Another way to apply cold involves freezing water in a disposable insulated coffee cup. The sides at the top are peeled away and the ice then rubbed gently over the skin until it becomes bright pink, usually 7 to 10 minutes. The container should be moved continuously to prevent frostbite and peeled away as the ice melts.

Compression

Edema is the sports physician's enemy for at least three reasons. It can form an insulating barrier keeping cold therapy from affecting deeper tissues; its presence around a joint can interfere with normal movement and hence the effectiveness of rehabilitative exercises; and, if there is tissue disruption, the edema can keep the ligament ends apart so that healing is with a fibrous scar rather than by ligament-to-ligament growth (Fig. 32). Fibrous scar healing can produce a ligament that is longer and therefore more lax than it was originally, so the joint is susceptible to reinjury when stressed. Elastic-bandage compression assists in minimizing the amount of edema and should be worn continuously for several days at least. Such external compression increases the hydrostatic pressure of the interstitial fluid and therefore counteracts the intravascular hydrostatic pressure and interstitial osmolarity, which cause fluid to move out of the capillaries into the interstitium. Compression is particularly difficult to apply consistently around the ankle, but this can be handled by padding the hollow between the malleoli and the Achilles tendon using felt pads or layered disposable diapers folded several times, cut into the shape of a horseshoe, and then placed around and inferior to each of the malleoli.

Elevation

Elevation of an injured limb reduces the hydrostatic pressure component of the forces driving plasma into the interstitium, and decreases the amount of edema by encouraging lymphatic drainage, especially if the injured part can be raised to at least the level of the heart.

Analgesics

Bleeding can persist even after minor trauma for at least several days after an injury. A single dose of aspirin (650 mg) can double the bleeding time for up to a week. As the breakdown of blood in the tissue causes further inflammation and edema, it does not seem rational to use aspirin, a known anticoagulant, as an analgesic for minor pain from soft-tissue injuries. As acetaminophen is considered to be equianalgesic to aspirin, this would appear to be the initial drug of choice. It is true that acetaminophen has little or no anti-inflammatory activity; however, the usual dose of aspirin given for pain relief has little or no anti-inflammatory activity either, something only achieved with the larger doses recommended for rheumatic fever and Kawasaki disease. At least one study has shown 50% greater postoperative swelling following molar tooth extractions when patients received aspirin compared to those who received acetaminophen.[3] These authors postulated that this might be due to aspirin-induced bleeding into the tissues. If acetaminophen is recommended, adult-sized adolescents will need to receive 650 mg qid.

Nonsteroidal anti-inflammatory drugs such as ibuprofen have a theoretical advantage over either acetaminophen or aspirin in being both anti-inflammatory and analgesic at the usual recommended doses. Many sports medicine specialists routinely prescribe anti-inflammatory drugs such as ibuprofen for most soft-tissue injuries in the belief that much of the body's inflammatory response to an injury is an "overreaction" that actually delays healing. At least one study has shown that this practice reduced pain and recovery time of injuries to the knee.[4]

*This chapter is reprinted by permission of *Pediatrics*. Dyment PG. Athletic Injuries. *Pediatrics in Review*. 1989;10:291-299

REFERENCES

1. American Academy of Orthopedic Surgeons. *Athletic Training and Sports Medicine*. Chicago, IL: American Academy of Orthopedic Surgeons; 1984
2. Hocutt JE, Jaffe R, Rylander CR, Beebe JK. Cryotherapy in ankle sprains. *Am J Sports Med*. 1982;10:316-319
3. Skjelbred P, Album B, Lokken P. Acetylsalicylic acid vs paracetemol: effects on postoperative course. *Eur J Clin Pharmacol*. 1977;12:257-264
4. Hutson MA. A double-blind study comparing ibuprofen, 1800 mg or 2400 mg daily, and placebo in sports injuries. *J Int Med Res*. 1986;14:142-147

Table 31. Severity of Strains and Sprains

Grade I   No appreciable disruption of tissue with a minimal loss of function ("mild").

Grade II   Moderate disruption of tissue with a partial loss of function ("moderate").

Grade III   Significant or complete disruption of tissue with a marked or complete loss of function ("severe").

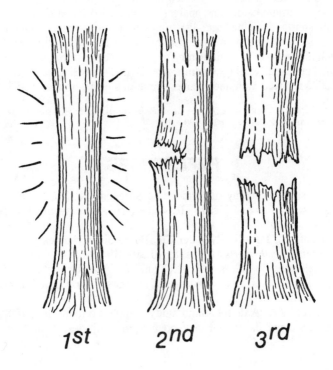

FIG. 29. Grades of Severity of Strains and Sprains.

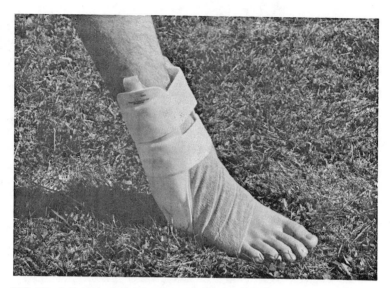

FIG. 30. Inflatable Splint for Ankle Sprain (Aircast).

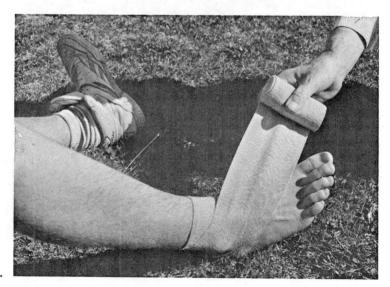

A.

FIG. 31. Cryotherapy for Ankle Sprain. A. Initial layer of wet bandage, B. ice chips in plastic bag applied to sprained area, C. ice left in place for 20 minutes.

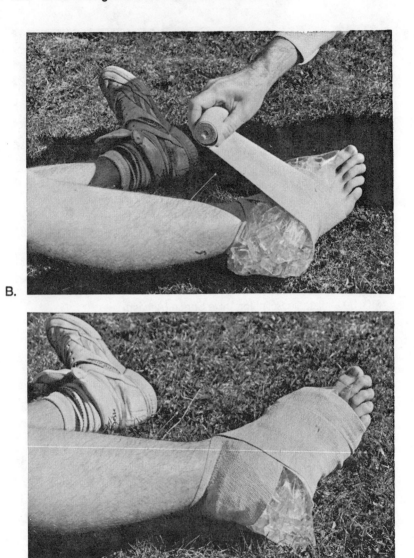

B.

C.

FIG. 31. *(continued)*

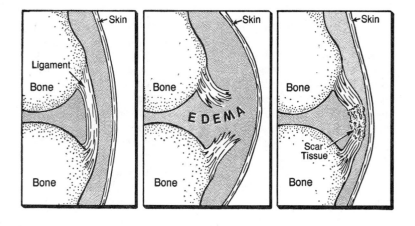

FIG. 32. Sprained Ligament Healing With Scar Tissue Producing a
Weaker and More Lax Ligament.

CHAPTER 17

FRACTURES AND DISLOCATIONS

The growing athlete sustains injuries that are different from those encountered in the skeletally mature athlete. The articular surfaces of the maturing athlete are increasing in size and changing in configuration, and possess different cellular characteristics. The growth plate (physis) is contributing to longitudinal growth. The periosteum is comparatively stronger and more cellularly active for peripheral growth and repair. The diaphysis (shaft) is more resilient, vascular, cellular, and porous.

The maturation of the entire epiphysis, which includes the articular surface, secondary ossification center of the epiphysis, and growing physis, provides a progressively changing pattern from cartilage to ossification. This growth pattern varies from bone to bone (Fig. 33). Many of the developmental lesions that occur in the young athlete–the so-called osteochondroses and overuse syndromes–are closely related to these biologic processes of growth and development. It is essential that all professional personnel dealing with school athletic programs understand the principles of musculoskeletal system growth and development. There are unique problems frequently ·associated with sports injuries in this population, as well as potential long-term implications from these injuries and developmental variants.

Fractures

A fracture is an interruption in the structure of a bone. The characteristics of the fracture are determined by the anatomic area affected and the forces causing the injury. In general, fractures of the metaphyseal area, a rich, cellular, and vascular cancellous bone, heal more rapidly than fractures of the diaphysis or cortical bone. Fractures of the epiphysis may heal rapidly. However, the potential for long-term modifications of growth is of significant concern.

Fractures are generally classified as closed or open (compound) fractures. If direct trauma has resulted in extensive skin and muscle damage with possible neurovascular compromise, a comprehensive treatment plan for bone stabilization, soft-tissue care, and potential infection will require the involvement of multiple consulting services. In some instances an open fracture may appear innocuous, such as a fracture associated with a small puncture wound. The puncture wound may be a result of an indirect force causing a severe angular deformity of the fractured bones and skin disruption from within. These are truly iceberg-like fractures, and the real concern is in the depths of the wound. To assess the potential for abscess, myonecrosis, and osteomyelitis, it is important to know what the tip of the bone has touched and what part of the exterior environment may have returned to the depths of the wound with the bone. Such fractures should be considered just as "open" as other direct "open" (compound) fractures with appropriate general wound care and the use of tetanus prophylaxis and antibiotics.

Whether a fracture is open or closed, the potential for a compartment syndrome should not be forgotten. Unrecognized compartment syndromes may result in significant loss of function and the potential loss of a limb. The hallmark symptoms of an impending compartment syndrome include extraordinary pain, swelling, pulse reduction, and sensory loss. Treatment should be implemented before loss of pulse, late sensory loss, and/or motor loss develop, as irreversible change and permanent functional impairment may follow these conditions. A compartment syndrome may be clinically suspected 12 to 24 hours postinjury and diagnosed at 24 to 36 hours postinjury; after 36 to 48 hours there is an increased likelihood of permanent residual impairment. If there is clinical suspicion of a compartment syndrome, immediate evaluation by intracompartmental pressure is necessary. If the diagnosis of a compartment syndrome is confirmed, an emergency surgical decompression must be planned.

The diagnosis of a fracture is obvious if there is significant deformity by clinical examination and/or supportive radiographic examination. However, there are times when diagnosis is much more difficult, eg, instances of lesser pain or nondisplaced fractures. An undisplaced fracture may not be obvious on initial conventional two-plane radiographs. Radiographs taken 7 to 14 days after an injury may show evidence of fracture and callus. The location of pain by careful digital evaluation may be the most valuable clinical diagnostic test, particularly in an athlete who has persistent pain and disability after primary radiographs have been interpreted as "no evidence of fracture." The most frequent examples of such undiagnosed, minimally displaced fractures are intra-articular fractures, epiphyseal fractures with primary cartilaginous involvement, and carpal or tarsal fractures. If there is clinical suspicion of a fracture, it is important to treat it as a fracture until additional evaluations, such as repeat radiographs, a technetium bone scan, CT scan, tomograms, or other image techniques provide significant supplemental information.

An undiagnosed fracture carries significant secondary concerns with parents, peers, and coaches. The most frequent undiagnosed fracture is the minimally displaced fracture of the distal fibular epiphysis. It is usually diagnosed as a severe ankle sprain. However, when the athlete cannot run at full speed 3 to 4 weeks postinjury, various concerns begin to surface. It is most unusual for an actively involved young athlete not to want to return to the competitive status. On the other hand, chronic pain is a frequent complaint for young athletes who seek to graciously leave an athletic situation that is not desirable for them. In many instances, it is difficult to differentiate the child seeking a gracious exit from the child with an undiagnosed fracture, particularly if the siblings or parents are encouraging the child to continue participation. Frequently, when the reason for the persistent pain is not quickly diagnosed, they will seek other consultations and may receive differing opinions that could confuse all concerned with the athlete's career.

The characteristics of a fracture as described by traditional terminology provide an implication of the location, healing potential, and possible long-term concerns. Frequently used fracture classifications in the pediatric age group include intra-articular, epiphyseal/physeal, avulsion, torus (buckle), diaphyseal (greenstick), stress, and pathologic fractures.

Intra-articular Fracture

An intra-articular fracture is one that extends through the articular surface and into the joint. There are many possible variations of fractures that would be termed intra-articular. They range from those that are entirely a fragment of cartilage, not visualized on radiograph, to fragments that are primarily cartilage with an osseous component that varies in size. The most serious of these is a fracture that extends from the metaphysis across the growth plate (physis) and the secondary ossification center of the epiphysis into the articular surface. Such a fracture carries the greatest potential for ultimate growth inhibition and associated intra-articular deformity. It is frequently necessary to operate on intra-articular fractures to reestablish normal joint surface continuity and provide articular surface congruity.

Osteochondritis dissecans connotes the development of an osteochondral fragment of articular cartilage on the underlying bone at the superficial surface of a diarthrodial joint. The osteochondral fragment may be in situ, incompletely detached, or completely detached and free within the joint. The clinical presentation is usually a complaint of arthralgia with an associated joint effusion. In more advanced cases, joint locking, instability, and/or articular degeneration may be observed. The patient is most frequently an adolescent male, and the joint most frequently affected is the knee, although involvement of the ankle, elbow, hip, and other diarthrodial joints has been observed. The diagnosis is suspected from historical and clinical examination, and is ultimately confirmed by the characteristic radiographic demarcation of a crescent-shaped area of radiolucency in the subchondral bone that may or may not appear to extend into the articular surface. A subchondral intra-articular fracture is evident if the area of radiolucency extends through the articular cartilage. The underlying bone pathology presents findings consistent with focal avascular osteonecrosis followed by repair or nonunion with occasional separation of the fragment. Recognition of the diagnosis and modified activity are the primary modes of treatment for the young athlete. Surgery, open or arthroscopic, is infrequently necessary.

Epiphyseal/Physeal Fracture

Injuries to epiphyseal areas are common in childhood. Approximately 10% to 15% of all skeletal trauma in childhood involves an epiphyseal injury. Of the total number of epiphyseal injuries, approximately 5% result in a variation of growth. The classification of epiphyseal injuries is usually recorded in the categories proposed by Salter and Harris (Fig. 34). In general, the more significant the force causing the fracture, the greater the likelihood of a secondary growth disturbance. The anatomic location of the epiphyseal fracture and the age of the individual will affect the prognosis. Obviously, the younger the child the more growth potential and the greater the possibility of a major deformity.

Growth disturbances may result in limb length discrepancies, intra-articular incongruities, and metaphyseal angular deformities. Limb length variances are not always evident soon after the fracture. In some instances, there may be a progressive retardation of growth prior to ultimate cessation. Therefore, the healing of a fracture on radiograph and the return of a child to normal activity should not be considered a terminal point for follow-up. The extremities should be measured and joint function observed at periodic visits for at least 2 years after an epiphyseal injury. If there is an alteration of growth or a deformity of the extremity, then appropriate radiographs of the affected and noninjured extremities must be compared. If an alteration of growth should occur, there are a number of surgical procedures that can be considered for correcting such deformities, including resection of a bone bridge across a physis, arrest of a physis (epiphyseodeses), corrective osteotomies, leg lengthenings, and leg shortenings. Additional problems are to be considered if the growth disturbance has occurred in one bone of a two-bone segment, ie, forearm (radius and ulna) or leg (tibia and fibula). In such instances, one bone will probably continue to grow at a normal rate, resulting in specific concerns regarding length and joint function.

A slipped capital femoral epiphysis may be considered a variant of an epiphyseal fracture and is usually diagnosed at the onset of rapid growth acceleration (Tanner 2 to 4) in children who are moderately obese or unusually tall for their stage of development. In some instances, there is a prodromal period of hip pain or referred hip pain to the knee, which may cause a limp after stressful activity. Many hip problems of childhood present as knee pain, a referred pain on the basis of associated obturator nerve innervation. The diagnosis of a slipped capital femoral epiphysis will require surgery. It should be noted that approximately 25% of individuals with a slipped epiphysis will show clinical evidence of a slipped capital femoral epiphysis on the contralateral side, at the same or later time, prior to completing skeletal growth.

Chronic overactivity may result in epiphyseal stress complaints with recurrent pain. This is most likely to occur in children who are limiting their activity to one sport and performing specific, repetitive actions on a frequent basis in that one sport. Some examples are distal femoral epiphyseal discomfort in young swimmers working on the breast-stroke kick, and shoulder discomfort in baseball or tennis players with repetitive stress about their shoulder. Treatment requires a period of rest or at least a modification of the usual frequency of the specific motion or activity. In general, the use of nonsteroidal anti-inflammatory medication is not necessary.

Avulsion Fracture

The major musculotendinous units are attached to bone through a structure very similar to an epiphysis. However, since it does not contribute to longitudinal growth, it is called an apophysis. The origin and insertion area is usually associated with a prominence or tubercle such as the patella tendon into the anterior tibial tubercle, the iliopsoas to the lesser trochanter of the femur, the origin of the sartorius from the anterior superior iliac spine, the hamstrings from the ischium, and the forearm flexors from the medial epicondyle of the humerus. These areas are particularly susceptible to an avulsion fracture during periods of rapid growth.

Sudden or repetitive contractile forces may result in an avulsion fracture: an acute or chronic separation of the apophysis. If the avulsion is primarily of the fibrocartilaginous portion, it may not be readily diagnosed at an early stage by radiograph. In most instances, a portion of bone is avulsed, or a callus may be seen radiographically, as in repetitive microinjury. A classic example of an acute avulsion fracture is an adolescent runner who suddenly feels a "pop" in the groin area, frequently described as a knife-like pain. This would be characteristic of an avulsion fracture of the iliopsoas insertion into the lesser trochanter. Examples of chronic repetitive avulsion fractures are "Little League elbow" due to repetitive forces on the medial epicondyle and Osgood-Schlatter's disease from repetitive forces of the patella tendon insertion into the anterior tibial tubercle. Usually a period of rest and progressive rehabilitation is sufficient, with a predictable, excellent result. It is a rare instance when any of the avulsion fractures require surgical intervention.

Torus or Buckle Fracture

If a symmetrical or asymmetrical longitudinal force is directed to the metaphyseal area of the bone, it may result in a compressive injury of the cancellous bone of the metaphysis. If it is equally distributed to the entire metaphysis, there will be a circumferential bulging in the bone of the metaphysis, resulting in a torus fracture. If the force is asymmetrical and localizes in one area, then it is more likely to be called a buckle fracture. The distal radius is the most common site for either the torus or buckle fracture. These fractures heal very rapidly because of their intrinsic stability, as well as the biology of the cellular metaphyseal bone. The symptoms are less severe than with most fractures. In general, a 2- to 3-week period of immobilization for comfort and protection against further injury is sufficient.

Diaphyseal (Greenstick) Fracture

Forces that are directed to the shaft of the bone may result in either a complete or incomplete fracture. In the growing child, the bone is more flexible and an incomplete fracture, known as a greenstick fracture, will occur. This terminology is derived from the radiographic appearance of a curved bone, an appearance similar to the bending of a sapling. In some instances there will be such extreme deformation that residual bowing is present without evidence of a major fracture. This is called plastic deformation. The most common site for a greenstick fracture is one of the bones of the forearm. It is necessary to realign the greenstick deformity to prevent a significant residual angular deformity, which can cause restriction of forearm rotation.

The classification of other diaphyseal fractures in children use the same terms as adult fractures, eg, spiral fracture, comminuted fracture, and transverse fracture. Many fractures in young athletes are likely to be spiral fractures of the tibia that remain in good position because of the strong periosteum. It is extraordinary for any child to require an open reduction of a diaphyseal fracture.

A concern that should be noted regarding diaphyseal fractures in children is the potential for a subsequent growth variance. An acceleration of growth is most frequent following fractures of the femur and, to a lesser degree, the tibia. It is not uncommon for a fracture of the femur in a growing child to result in an overgrowth of 1 to 2 cm. On occasion, if major longitudinal forces cause the diaphyseal fracture, there may be a compressive injury to an epiphysis resulting in a later retardation or cessation of growth. The effect on growth may not be observed until visits 1 to 2 years postinjury. Thus, the child's growth pattern and spine examination should be monitored at annual intervals. If there is evidence of asymmetrical growth or scoliosis in a child who has had a diaphyseal fracture, orthopedic evaluation should be suggested.

Stress Fracture

Stress fractures are usually incomplete fractures that are most common in the bones of the feet and legs. They are frequently associated with repetitive activity that focuses a stress on a particular area of a bone. These were originally recognized as march fractures, identified in Army recruits who complained of severe foot pain in their early days of training. They were later known as fatigue fractures, implying a failure to tolerate stress. They are most common in the pediatric population in two situations: (1) when children have been relatively inactive during the summer suddenly become involved in a vigorous fall sport training program and complain of excruciating leg pain after 2 to 3 weeks; and when children remain active at a high level of demand, such as doing gymnastics or year-round running.

The recognition of stress fractures is primarily by suspicion from history and confirmation by either conventional radiograph or a technetium bone scan. An early-stage radiograph is frequently not diagnostic, whereas a technetium bone scan may be diagnostic. The differential diagnosis is tendinitis, stress periostitis, or various compartment syndromes. The treatment for stress fracture is usually a modification of activity: a limited participation in the sport that has resulted in the stress fracture for 6 to 12 weeks. Immobilization is infrequently necessary, and surgery is rarely required.

Pathologic Fracture

Metabolic bone diseases, benign tumors, and malignant tumors of children are frequently first noticed because of athletic injury. The progressive weakening of an area of the bone by these conditions will result in a greater susceptibility to fracture with minimal force: a pathologic fracture. A benign bone cyst is the most frequent cause of pathologic fracture in an athletic, healthy child. A fracture of the humerus by the vigorous throwing of a ball may be the initial indication of a bone lesion or osteogenesis imperfecta. The recurrent aching about a knee may be the presenting complaint for a malignant bone tumor. The initial awareness and suspicion of such potential diagnoses secondary to minor trauma are confirmed by characteristic observations on the radiograph and supplemental clinical and laboratory evaluations. The treatment and recommendations are determined by the specific diagnosis.

Dislocations

The movable joints of extremities are synovial, diarthrodial articulations. This classification implies joint surfaces of articular cartilage, intra-articular ligaments and menisci, a synovial lining, joint capsule, and periarticular ligaments and musculotendinous structures. A joint is dislocated if the articular surfaces are totally apart from one another. A joint is subluxed if the articular surfaces are partly separated. If the damage to intra-articular ligaments or menisci results in abnormal function, such as clicking, locking, or catching, the joint is internally deranged or functionally unstable.

Dislocations secondary to trauma are uncommon in the skeletally immature athletic population. In most instances where a joint appears dislocated, with the exception of a patella dislocation, it is more likely to be an epiphyseal fracture. Dislocations, especially of the fingers, toes, or shoulders, are more common in the skeletally mature athlete. In the mature group, early on-site reduction is usually indicated. In the skeletally immature athlete, it is important to have accurate radiographic evaluation prior to attempting manipulation in what appears to be a dislocation.

There are some individuals who have excessive ligamentous laxity and/or congenital muscle weakness who subluxate or dislocate their joints with minimal trauma. These are most unusual problems and require specific consultation to determine whether they should participate in sports. If so, they require external supportive devices. If their ability to subluxate or dislocate their joints is voluntary, there may be a need for psychiatric evaluation.

If a child does not have a dislocated joint and requires a manipulative reduction, it is important to observe the continued development of that joint and the growth of the bone during the period of growth. There may be impaired vascular dynamics to the entire epiphysis, which could result in avascular necrosis of a portion of the bone, such as the head of the femur or head of the humerus. Sufficient trauma to cause a dislocation could result in sufficient damage to interfere with normal growth potential. Again, long-term observation of the injured area is necessary. An early return to sports does not assure long-term normal function and growth. Gradual discomfort, limping, impairment of motion, and asymmetrical growth are clinical alert signals that require additional evaluation.

SUGGESTED READING

Blount WP. *Fractures in Children*. Melbourne, FL: Krieger Publishing; 1955

Rang M. *Children's Fractures*. 2nd ed. Philadelphia, PA: JB Lippincott; 1982

Rockwood CA Jr, Wilkins KE, King RE. *Fractures in Children*. Philadelphia, PA: JB Lippincott; 1984:vol 3

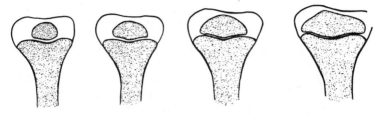

FIG. 33. Diagram Illustrating the Progressive Maturation of the Entire Epiphysis.

From Pappas AM. Epiphyseal injuries in sports. *Phys Sportsmed.* 1983;11(6):140-148. Reprinted by permission of *The Physician and Sportsmedicine.* Copyright McGraw-Hill, Inc.

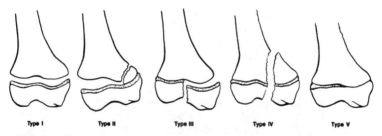

FIG. 34. Illustration of the Salter-Harris Classification of Epiphyseal Injuries.

From Pappas AM. Epiphyseal injuries in sports. *Phys Sportsmed.* 1983;11(6):140-148. Reprinted by permission of *The Physician and Sportsmedicine.* Copyright McGraw-Hill, Inc.

CHAPTER 18

ACUTE KNEE INJURIES

Knee injuries are common in football and account for the most common serious injuries in that sport. It has been estimated that during each week of the fall football season at least 6,000 high school and college players injure their knees, 10% of whom will require surgery! Even more discouraging are the results of a 20-year follow-up study of men who had sustained knee injuries in high school football. Thirty-nine percent still had significant symptoms, and 50% of these men had radiographic abnormalities.

Physicians attending football games should be familiar with the on-the-field management and diagnostic tests to perform on a player who suffers an acute knee injury.

The best time to examine an injured knee is immediately after the injury. Within an hour of a knee injury, protective muscle spasm can prevent a reliable assessment of the degree of the joint instability; the following day there may be enough of a joint effusion to preclude a satisfactory examination then as well. In the initial examination of an injured knee, preferably done on the field, one looks for gross ligamentous instability and osteochondral fractures. If there is any evidence of ligamentous injury, the athlete should not return to play that game. If there is significant laxity of one of the collateral ligaments, most primary care physicians will refer the patient to an orthopedic surgeon who will perform more comprehensive testing.

On-the-Field Examination

1. A fracture should be excluded by questioning, observing, and testing for severe localized pain, deformity, and an inability to bear weight. A young athlete could have an epiphyseal fracture evident only by pain at that site when a varus or valgus stress is applied.
2. Perform an anterior drawer test with the knee in 30° of flexion (Lachman test) (Fig. 35). The injured leg is externally rotated slightly to relax the hamstrings and adductor muscles. The examiner kneels lateral to the injured leg, stabilizes the femur with one hand, and directs a gentle but firm upward force with the other hand on the proximal tibia. If the tibia moves anteriorly, the anterior cruciate ligament has been torn.
3. Without moving your hands, a posterior force is applied to the tibia, and, if there is posterior movement, the posterior cruciate ligament

has been injured.

4. Then perform an abduction/adduction stress test with the knee still at 30° flexion (Fig. 36). The integrity of the medial collateral ligament (MCL) is assessed by applying a valgus stress by holding the tibia about a third of the way down and forcing it gently laterally (abduction) while holding the distal femur in place. Some examiners use their thumb as a fulcrum to the lateral knee joint (Fig. 37). If there is an increased medial opening at the joint, the MCL has been damaged, although the medial capsular structures will probably also have been damaged. If the opening of the medial joint is large (more than 1 cm), damage to the anterior and posterior cruciate ligaments may also have occurred. If the only physical sign is acute pain in the area of the MCL, that ligament has probably sustained just a mild sprain.

5. The adductor test for determining lateral collateral ligament laxity is then done after moving to the other side of the player and repeating the test as above but applying a varus stress. Varus laxity with the knee in 30° flexion indicates that the lateral collateral ligament (and capsular structures) have been injured, and, as with the medial test, openings of 1 cm or more suggest involvement of the cruciate ligaments.

Medial Collateral Ligament

The most common knee injury is a sprain of the MCL. This important ligament is the medial stabilizer of the knee, and it is usually injured by a direct blow to the lateral aspect of the knee. The resulting valgus (medial) stress can result in a Grade I, II, or III sprain (see Chapter 16). The player is usually able to bear some weight on the leg immediately after the injury, and players have been known to actually continue playing despite a Grade III sprain. Medial knee pain is usually felt at the time of the injury, and the knee may feel "wobbly" while the player walks afterwards.

The examination will reveal acute tenderness somewhere over the course of the MCL, usually at or above the joint line. If the knee is being examined several hours after the injury, there may be swelling and ecchymosis over the ligament, or sometimes even a joint effusion. Pain over the ligament or separation of the medial joint when performing the abductor stress test indicates that this is the most likely diagnosis.

A first-degree sprain of this ligament is treated with rest, ice, compression, and elevation (see Chapter 16), and running should be restricted until the athlete has pain-free knee flexion. Generally, in 5 to 10 days, there will be a completely recovered range of motion without pain, and, if the athlete can perform all the movements required in that sport without pain and has been examined by a physician, he or she can return to full activity. The management of more serious sprains should be directed by an orthopedist.

Anterior Cruciate Ligament

A torn anterior cruciate ligament is the most common severe ligamentous injury to the knee. It usually occurs without an external force being applied, but rather when the athlete changes direction while running, and suddenly the knee "gives out." A pop will be felt, and the player goes down on the field and is unable to continue playing. A bloody effusion will slowly develop in the next 24 hours if there has been a severe injury, one more reason why knee injuries need to be examined right away. Young athletes with signs suggesting a torn anterior cruciate ligament require prompt referral to an orthopedic surgeon.

Meniscus Injuries

The practitioner should be aware of meniscal injuries when evaluating the athlete with an acute knee injury. They may occur following a twisting impact to the knee, or hyperflexion or hyperextension. The medial meniscus is attached to the medial collateral ligament and is frequently damaged along with that ligament when a tackle is directed towards the lateral side of the knee producing external rotation of the tibia (rupturing the medial meniscus) and also stretching the medial collateral ligament producing a sprain.

The following findings are generally present when one of the menisci (usually the medial) is damaged: (1) there is tenderness over the medial or lateral joint line, which should be differentiated from tenderness along the entire MCL elicited when that ligament is sprained; (2) there is pain at the medial or lateral joint line on hyperextension or hyperflexion of the knee; and (3) when the lower leg is rotated and the knee is flexed about 90°, pain during external rotation indicates a medial meniscus injury, whereas internal rotation produces pain with a lateral meniscus injury.

Dislocation of the Patella

This injury can result from a blow to the patella or when an athlete changes direction ("cutting") and then straightens the leg. The dislocation usually occurs laterally, but the medial joint capsule and retinaculum are also torn, sometimes simulating an MCL ligament sprain, if not actually associated with one. The dislocation usually reduces spontaneously, and the athlete will have a painful swollen knee (due to hemarthrosis) and tenderness at the medial capsule. Lateral pressure on the patella while gently extending the knee will be met with obvious anxiety and resistance. If this diagnosis is suspected, the leg should be splinted, and the athlete should be transported to a hospital for an examination by an orthopedist.

SUGGESTED READING

Zarins B, Admas M. Knee injuries in sports. *N Engl J Med.* 1988;318:950-961

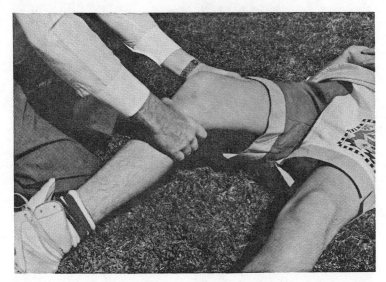

FIG. 35. Drawer Test for Anterior and Posterior Movement (Lachman Test).

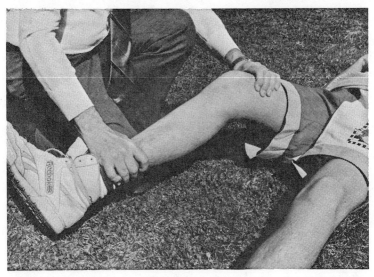

FIG. 36. Abduction Stress Test for Medial Collateral Ligament Sprain.

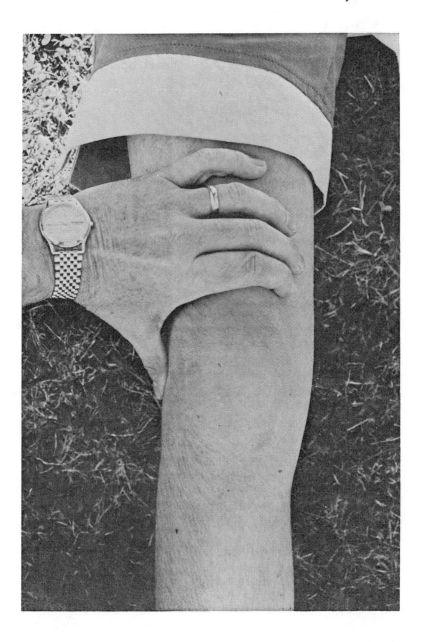

FIG. 37. Thumb Being Used as a Fulcrum When Performing Stress Test.

CHAPTER 19

HEAD AND NECK INJURIES[1]

Head Injuries

Epidemiology

It has been estimated that one in five high school football players suffers a concussion each season, resulting in over 250,000 concussions each year in this sport alone![2] The far less common life-threatening injuries are almost always subdural hematomas. In 1984, 16 high school athletes, fewer than 2 per 100,000 participants, had intracranial hematomas; six subsequently died. Head injuries account for approximately two thirds of all deaths in football.[3]

Although incidence figures are less available for other sports, head injury occurs occasionally in the following: baseball, from pitched balls or thrown bats; golf, from thrown clubs or hit balls; recreational bicycling, from falls or collisions with cars; horseback-riding, from falls or kicks; recreational diving, from hitting the bottom of the pool; boxing and wrestling; vehicular sports; all collision and contact sports, such as the martial arts, field hockey, ice hockey, soccer, and basketball; and noncontact activities, such as gymnastics and racquet sports.[4-7]

Kinds of Injuries

Concussion

The most common significant head injury in sports is concussion, a transient impairment of neural function caused by head trauma. Associated symptoms may include dizziness, headache, tinnitus, blurred vision, diplopia, confusion, loss of consciousness, amnesia, lack of awareness, drowsiness, nausea, vomiting, or hallucination.

The presence of amnesia is important both in indicating that concussion has occurred and in revealing its severity. With anterograde (post-traumatic) amnesia, the athlete cannot acquire, interpret, or retain new information, including the memory of events just subsequent to the injury. This inability may persist for a few minutes or for several hours.[8] On occasion, anterograde amnesia may take 3 to 20 minutes to develop.[9] Retrograde amnesia has two manifestations. First, there may be memory loss for events occurring several years before the injury; this lessens within several hours and eventually disappears. Second, there may be memory loss for events occurring seconds to minutes before the injury, and this memory loss persists. The presence of retrograde amnesia indicates a more serious injury than does isolated anterograde amnesia.[8-10]

Various schemes for grading the severity of concussions have been devised, but here they will be described as mild, moderate, or severe (Table 32), as recommended by Cantu.[10] Both the duration of loss of consciousness and of anterograde amnesia are used to determine the severity.

With mild concussions, which account for more than 50% of these injuries, athletes do not lose consciousness. They will be temporarily dazed and confused and may have mild gait abnormalities. In their vernacular, they may say that they were "dinged." Anterograde amnesia, if present, persists for less than 30 minutes. Occasionally, these athletes will have retrograde amnesia or other symptoms such as headache or dizziness.

A moderate concussion involves loss of consciousness, but for less than 5 minutes, or anterograde amnesia lasting more than 30 minutes but less than 24 hours. Retrograde amnesia is frequently present, and symptoms such as headache and nausea are common.

In a severe concussion, loss of consciousness lasts for at least 5 minutes, or anterograde amnesia lasts for at least 24 hours. This degree of injury is frequently caused by a frank intracranial hemorrhage evident on computed tomographic (CT) scan.

Postconcussion syndrome

A common complication of concussion is the postconcussion syndrome. In adolescents, its symptoms include recurrent headache and dizziness, especially with exertion; irritability, fatigue, and other personality changes; and difficulty with concentration, memory, and other higher integrative functions. Children may exhibit behavioral changes such as aggressiveness, disobedience, regressive behavior, and anxiety. Persistence of the syndrome for more than several days indicates that the athlete may need a CT scan or magnetic resonance imaging (MRI) and neuropsychiatric evaluation. Athletes should not return to full activity until all symptoms are gone.[8,10]

Life-threatening complications of head injury

A complete discussion of these is beyond the scope of this article, but the physician must be aware of the clinical presentations of the rare life-threatening complications of head injury. Most involve intracranial hemorrhage. The most common injury in sports causing death is a subdural hematoma, in which blood accumulates in a localized area beneath the dura mater, causing increased intracranial pressure. The athlete may be unconscious from the time of injury, or else awaken with subsequent deterioration, developing symptoms such as headache, nausea, and vomiting.

In an epidural hematoma, the blood is external to the dura. This injury usually occurs when a hard, localized blow fractures the temporal bone, tearing the underlying middle meningeal artery. Typically the athlete has a brief lucid interval, with symptoms beginning 10 to 15 minutes, but sometimes hours, later. The expanding hemorrhage causes headache, nausea, and vomiting. Pressure on the adjacent frontal cortex may cause weakness in the face and arm on the opposite side.

In an intracerebral hematoma, there is hemorrhage into the brain itself. This is the usual cause of death in boxers who do not regain consciousness after a knockout.

Cerebral hyperemia is a consequence of head injury occasionally seen in children, almost always in individuals less than 16 years old. Generalized dilation of cerebral vessels causes increased intracranial pressure. It occurs within minutes to hours of injury. If a lucid interval precedes it, its presentation mimics that of an intracranial hematoma. The prognosis is good if the associated traumatic brain injury is not severe[11] and the athlete receives proper management for increased intracranial pressure.

Posttraumatic migraine

Head trauma may cause an attack of migraine within minutes to hours of the injury. The symptoms (for example, confusion, aphasia, hemiparesis, headache, nausea, and vomiting) can obviously be confused with those resulting from significant brain injury. The diagnosis may be less apparent in those who have neurologic symptoms without headache. The precipitating injury is usually a mild concussion. The athlete may have had a similar previous episode with or without head trauma.[12,13]

Clinical Evaluation

Preparation

Adults working with young athletes must be prepared for the possibility of severe head and neck injury. Proper preparation includes designating the person who will be in charge of on-the-field management; ensuring the availability of proper emergency medical equipment, especially that needed for cardiopulmonary resuscitation (CPR); training all supervising adults in CPR and in the handling of athletes with head and neck injuries; selecting an ambulance service with appropriate equipment, including a spineboard and a properly trained staff; choosing a hospital with neurosurgical treatment facilities; and knowing the location of a nearby telephone with which emergency help can be summoned.[14]

With any head injury, the possibility of cervical spine injury must be considered. This will be discussed more completely later in this chapter.

On-the-field evaluation

Mild concussions may be hard to recognize, particularly if the head injury was not observed. Affected athletes at times may be identified because they appear dazed or confused or cannot remember what they are supposed to be doing. Athletes with suspected mild concussions should be removed from play. They should be evaluated for the presence of anterograde amnesia with such questions as who helped them to their feet, how they got to the sidelines, and what is the first thing they can remember after being hit. During the evaluation, the examiner should note their ability to understand and respond to the questions. They may exhibit perseverative questioning about recent events. Athletes should be evaluated for retrograde amnesia with questions such as what happened at the moment of injury and what they were doing just before it —for example, whether they were playing offense or defense and the number of the player they were guarding. Their orientation to person, place, and time should be determined. They must also be questioned about neurologic symptoms such as headache and dizziness.[8,10]

If an athlete loses consciousness, the evaluator should ensure that pulse and respirations are normal. If so, the athlete should be left alone to awaken. A significant neck injury should be assumed to be present until proven otherwise. The head should be held by hand (see neck injury discussion). No other manipulation should occur. A football player should not have his chin strap and helmet removed. If the athlete awakens within several seconds, the evaluator should establish whether a neck injury is present (see neck injury discussion). If this can be effectively ruled out, the athlete can be removed from the game and evaluated at a medical facility. If neck injury cannot be ruled out, or if unconsciousness lasts for more than several seconds, the athlete should be carefully moved onto a spineboard and transported to a hospital with neurosurgical treatment facilities. Unless the adults present have the proper equipment and expertise, the athlete should not be moved until emergency medicine technicians arrive with an ambulance.[14] Athletes with severe concussions should be evaluated at the medical facility for possible intracranial bleeding.

If a seizure occurs and the tongue appears to be obstructing the airway, the athlete should be rolled onto the side, with precautions taken to keep the neck in proper alignment. Gravity will usually bring the tongue forward and out of the way. Nothing should be inserted into the mouth "to keep the athlete from biting the tongue"; this previously recommended practice is now believed to be unnecessary and likely to cause injury.

Return to Competition

The following guidelines have been developed with the help of several child neurologists and neurosurgeons and after reviewing the literature, particularly the excellent article by Cantu.[10] It is impossible to find unanimity on this subject. These are only guidelines and individual circumstances must be taken into account.

The physician should be aware of the "second impact syndrome," in which fatal cerebral edema results from a second minor head injury that follows a recent episode of apparently minor head trauma. Some but not all individuals who experience this problem have an unrecognized mass lesion from the initial episode. This syndrome is rare, but a successful lawsuit has been brought against at least one physician who was unaware of it.[10,15] It is one of several reasons for which athletes should not return to play after a head injury until they are symptom-free, and why it is best to be more, rather than less, conservative in return-to-play decisions. There is research suggesting that concussions may cause cumulative, permanent brain injury.[16] At the very least, it appears that recovery of high cognitive functions and disappearance of minor neurologic symptoms may take several months if a second concussion occurs soon after the first.[17]

The following guidelines are rather liberal. Some neurologists and neurosurgeons would advocate greater conservatism.

An athlete at the junior high school level or below who has experienced a mild concussion should not return to play that day even if full recovery occurs within minutes. After 15 to 30 minutes of observation, a high school or college athlete may return to play if, at rest, there is no headache, dizziness, impaired concentration, inability to understand and retain information (anterograde amnesia), lack of orientation to time, person, and place, or retrograde amnesia, and, with exertion, the athlete must remain symptom-free and be able to perform the maneuvers of the sport with usual skill. Otherwise, the athlete can return the following day if all symptoms are gone both at rest and upon exertion.[10] If headache or other symptoms worsen in the first 24 hours or last for more than a week, a complete neurologic examination and CT scan or MRI is probably indicated.[10]

After a moderate concussion, the athlete can return 7 days after all symptoms are gone at rest and during exercise. Behavior and school performance must be normal, and an examination by a physician is required.[10]

After a severe concussion, the athlete cannot return to participation for at least one month. All neurologic symptoms must have been absent for at least one week, behavior and school performance must be as before, and an examination by a physician is necessary. An abnormality on CT scan or MRI such as an intracranial hematoma indicates that the athlete should not participate in any further play during that season.[10]

If a young athlete experiences a second concussion during the same season, even if it is mild, more restrictive rules apply (Table 33). For example, two severe concussions should terminate contact sports until the next season. The circumstances of the injuries must also be reviewed carefully because prevention may be possible. For example, a football player who is contacting the runner with his head when tackling ("spearing") should avoid this dangerous technique.[10]

If the young athlete seems to be at particular risk of another injury, eg, a small athlete playing a collision sport against bigger players, termination of the season or a switch to a safer sport may be advisable after the first concussion. Because the retention and processing of information is often significantly affected even with mild concussions, athletes in certain dangerous sports such as automobile racing may need to wait longer than others before they return to competition.[10]

Athletes who have had surgical or other major complications of head injury should not return to full participation until their supervising physician approves. The decision concerning return to a high-risk sport should be individualized, but great caution should be exercised in allowing return to collision sports such as football and ice hockey.

Prevention

Several interventions can reduce the likelihood of head injury. In football, athletes who are tackling or being tackled must avoid making contact with their heads.[3] Helmets must have a stamp of approval by the National Operating Committee on Standards for Athletic Equipment (NOCSAE) and must fit well and be in good condition.[18] Unfortunately, relatively little attention is usually paid to the fit and the state of repair of athletes' helmets.

In baseball and softball, the catcher, batter, and base runner should wear protective helmets. Bicyclists should be taught to wear helmets and to observe safety rules.[20] Prevention among swimmers is discussed below in the section on neck injuries. Horseback riders, particularly those involved in steeplechase, jumping, and flat racing, should wear helmets, as should ice hockey players.

The American Academy of Pediatrics has recommended the elimination of boxing (Appendix 6), but as it continues, pediatricians should work to eliminate boxing among their patients and in their communities.

Neck Injuries
Epidemiology

In sports, serious cervical spine injuries occur most often during recreational diving in shallow water.[21] Other sports with risk include water skiing, surf boarding, rugby, football, ice hockey, recreational bicycle riding, gymnastics, tumbling, horseback riding, wrestling, organized diving, snow skiing, scuba diving, weight lifting and training, the martial arts, and all other contact sports.[3-7,21] Serious injuries are less common in athletes less than 12 years of age compared to older adolescents.[4]

In 1984, 36 high school football players, or almost four per 100,000 participants, experienced fractures, dislocations, or subluxations of the cervical spine. Four became quadriplegic (about the same number each year for the past few years). These injuries most often occur in players who are executing tackles. Neck injuries cause approximately 20% of deaths in football. There has been a dramatic decrease in the incidence of these injuries since 1976 when "spearing," the use of the top of the head as a point of contact in blocking and tackling, was made illegal.[18] One report from Ontario has shown that ice hockey is more likely than football to produce quadriplegia.[19]

Athletes can sustain catastrophic neck injuries using a trampoline or minitrampoline, even if they are experienced and have spotters to catch them.[6] This has led the American Academy of Pediatrics to recommend that they *not* be used in routine physical education classes, at home, for recreation, nor as a competitive sport (Appendix 4).

Serious injuries leading to quadriplegia are almost always caused by axial compression of the spine when force is applied to the top of the head with the neck in flexion. Transmitted forces cause fractures or dislocations.[18]

Kinds of Injuries

Most kinds of athletic injuries to the cervical spine are described below. Only a small fraction of these result in permanent neurologic damage. In those that do, probably half result from improper handling of an athlete with an unstable injury.[18]

Neurapraxia of the brachial plexus

This injury (called a "burner" or a "stinger") is common in football players. It occurs when the neck is forced laterally, sometimes with rotation or anterior or posterior displacement. This injury pinches or stretches cervical nerve roots or the nerves of the upper brachial plexus.

The athlete feels sharp burning pain in the neck that may radiate into the shoulder and down the arm to the hand. There may be weakness and paresthesias in the involved area. The symptoms typically last seconds to minutes, sometimes longer. Neck pain, except transiently, is not an expected part of this syndrome. It is occasionally complicated by peripheral degeneration in nerves of the brachial plexus.[22,23]

Cervical strain

Cervical muscle strain is probably the commonest neck injury in sports. Bleeding and inflammation in the muscles cause local pain, and tenderness is located over the affected vertebrae. Limitation of motion is frequent. The athlete will often say he has "jammed" his neck.[22,23] The pain may not be significant initially but worsens as inflammation develops. The neurologic examination is normal, and no neurologic symptoms will be reported.[22,23]

Serious injuries

Axial compression-flexion injuries may disrupt the posterior soft tissues stabilizing the cervical spine, causing vertebral subluxation without fracture. Pain over the cervical vertebrae in the area of injury will usually be present, but the neurologic examination will be normal. No fractures will be seen on x-rays. The injury is identified on lateral flexion-extension views, which show instability. They may not be obtainable until acute inflammation and secondary limitation of motion have subsided.[22,23] Hence, in neck injuries, these views should be repeated once range of motion has returned to normal.

Cervical fractures and dislocations also usually result from axial compression with flexion. They may be stable or unstable, and neurologic deficit may be present or absent.[22,23] An occasional athlete may complain of burning paresthesias or dysesthesias in his hands beginning at the moment of injury, usually, but not always, associated with neck pain.[24] The unstable injuries may result in worsening neurologic injury if the athlete's neck is not properly stabilized when he is moved.

Not only may vertebral subluxation not be demonstrable on initial radiographs, but there are other serious injuries in which radiographs may be normal. One is a ruptured cervical intervertebral disk. Second, in athletes less than 16 years old, transient deformation of the cervical spine can permanently damage the cord without producing demonstrable injury, even subluxation, with imaging techniques. Some of these children, if questioned carefully, will report transient paresthesias, clumsiness, a subjective feeling of paralysis at the moment of injury, or the sensation of lightning running down the back of the legs. The onset of persistent symptoms is often delayed for minutes to days, and probably can be prevented in at least a few children by timely immobilization to prevent further damage from an unstable injury.[25,26]

Neck injury may occasionally cause transient quadriplegia with weakness or complete paralysis. Called "cervical spinal cord neurapraxia with transient quadriplegia," this injury is apparently caused by transient pressure of bony structures against the spinal cord that does not result in permanent injury. Sensory symptoms include burning paresthesias or loss of sensation. Neck pain is limited to burning paresthesia. Complete recovery usually occurs within 15 minutes, although rarely it requires 36 to 48 hours. These patients should be evaluated by a neurologist or neurosurgeon for underlying abnormalities of the cervical spine.[27]

Note two facts in the above discussion. Neck pain is usually, but not always, present in severe cervical spine injuries. Neurologic symptoms, even if transient, may indicate a serious injury and should be taken seriously.

Clinical Evaluation

On-the-field evaluation

Although they are rare, unstable fractures and dislocations of the cervical spine can lead to worsening neurologic injury or death if the athlete is improperly moved. This discussion will not deal with the details of cardiopulmonary resuscitation or proper transport, which are available in several sources.[14,22,23,28] It will describe general principles of evaluation and first aid. (See also the "Clinical Evaluation" section above in the discussion of head injuries.)

If a downed athlete has a possible cervical spine injury, the neck should immediately be stabilized between the hands of an adult who exerts gentle longitudinal traction. The next step is to evaluate, and, if necessary, open the airway. Often removing the mouthpiece is all that is needed. In athletes whose heads are turned or who are prone, proper technique in changing their position is essential. A football helmet should not be removed nor should the chin strap be loosened. The facemask can be removed if CPR is necessary, using bolt cutters (old style face mask) or a sharp knife or scalpel (new style). Head and neck motion during CPR should be minimized. Special training is required to prepare the coaches in a sports program to accomplish these maneuvers properly.[14,23,28] Such training is recommended, but few coaches probably have received it. It may never be needed, but may be lifesaving on rare occasions.

An unconscious athlete should be assumed to have a neck injury. Smelling salts should not be used because sudden motion of the neck as the athlete awakens might cause severe spinal cord damage. An ambulance should be summoned.

For athletes who are conscious, a rapid initial neurologic assessment is possible. The first step is to establish their ability to give an accurate history. They must be oriented to time, person, and place, and able to respond to questions and commands. They must report any paresthesias or feelings of paralysis. These, even if transient, imply serious cervical injury, and proper immobilization and transportation are the next steps. If these symptoms are absent, players should be asked to move fingers, toes, and all extremities. If this is possible, they then can use large muscle groups to push against the examiner's hand. Unilateral weakness in the upper or lower extremity can thus be identified.[14,23,28]

If the neurologic examination is normal, the next step is the examination of the neck. If there is pain at rest, immobilization is needed. If not, the athlete can make gentle voluntary motions against the examiner's hand in all directions. If this causes severe pain, the neck is immobilized. If pain is minimal or absent, the player can attempt gentle active motion. Severe pain again dictates immobilization. If there is little or no pain, the athlete can sit or stand up. If there is full range of neck motion and no more than mild pain at the extremes of motion, the player can leave the field.[28]

Active range of motion is evaluated by having the athlete nod the head, touch the chin to the chest, touch the chin to the right and left shoulder, and touch each ear to the adjacent shoulder. These movements should not be forced if they are painful.[14]

Proper immobilization and transport requires several trained individuals and appropriate equipment. If these are not available at the field, the athlete with apparent significant injury should be left alone until trained personnel arrive with the ambulance, unless CPR is needed.

In an athlete, usually a football player, with apparent brachial plexus neurapraxia, the sensation, strength, and reflexes in the affected arm must be evaluated.[14,23,28] Muscle strength should be tested in the shoulder rotators, deltoid, biceps, triceps, and forearm. The player should be questioned about the presence of persistent neck pain, which may indicate a more serious injury.

Cervical sprains and strains are relatively common, and unstable fractures and dislocations are rare. The experienced team physician or athletic trainer will not send every athlete with a neck injury to the emergency room on a spineboard. Many will be stabilized in a stiff cervical collar and sent for radiographs by car, or even diagnosed as having a muscle strain without x-rays. Until this experience is gained, or in confusing situations, the responsible adult should be overly conservative. Use of a spineboard should be considered, or at least a neck immobilizer. Radiographs should be performed on any athlete who has pain or limitation of motion, especially if the neck was injured in a collision. Transient or persistent neurologic symptoms also warrant x-rays, except in athletes with transient brachial plexus neurapraxia.

Radiographs

After clinical evaluation, the athlete with a possible significant neck injury on arrival at a treatment facility needs anterior/posterior (AP) and lateral cervical spinal radiographs to evaluate the vertebrae and adjacent soft tissues. The neck must not be moved until the radiologist is certain that there is no unstable fracture or dislocation. If possible, the films should be made using the equipment in the radiology department rather than portable equipment, which gives poorer resolution. The lateral view is followed by two AP views, one to visualize C3 to C7 and an open-mouth view for C1 to C2. Fluoroscopy or tomography may be necessary to visualize parts of vertebrae that are superimposed on others. The examination is incomplete until all seven cervical vertebrae are seen in two views. Myelography, CT, or MRI may be needed if the initial evaluation is inconclusive. Right and left oblique views are part of a complete evaluation. If all these radiographs are normal, lateral views in maximum voluntary flexion and extension are obtained to evaluate ligamentous integrity. Acute limitation of motion may require that these be repeated once full range of motion has been reestablished.[26]

Return to Play

Return to play following brachial plexus neurapraxia is permissible if strength, sensation, and reflexes are normal within a few minutes of injury, and persistent neck pain is absent. Symptoms lasting longer than this, particularly for more than 1 to 2 hours, or recurrence of this injury, even if symptoms are brief, both require x-rays and careful clinical evaluation by a neurologist or neurosurgeon before return to play.[14,23,28] The following recommendations for athletes with other injuries are a more conservative version of those suggested by Torg.[23]

After cervical spinal neurapraxia with transient quadriplegia, those athletes with instability or acute or chronic degenerative changes should avoid sports with risk of neck injury. Those with spinal stenosis should be considered individually, but great caution should be used since risk of recurrent problems is present in at least some.

Athletes with cervical sprains can return to full participation when they have a complete, pain-free range of cervical motion, no other symptoms, normal muscle strength, and no instability on flexion/extension x-rays. Reinjury is common, however. Individuals with disk injuries or stable wedge compression fractures should give up contact sports forever.

Those with subluxation without fracture should avoid contact sports forever, as should those who have had a cervical fusion. They may be able to return to other activities.

Prevention

Many injuries could probably be avoided with better conditioning of young athletes, better coaching in technique, improved supervision of practices, stricter enforcement of safety rules, and intolerance of foul play.

The prevention of injury in football has been discussed in the section on head injury. In addition, strengthening of the neck muscles is important. Athletes who have recurrent brachial plexus neurapraxia should have a strengthening program for their neck and shoulder muscles and wear a cervical collar when playing.[23] Swimmers should be taught not to dive into water that is shallower than twice their height.[5] In ice hockey, rules must be carefully enforced, especially those against boarding, cross-checking, pushing, or checking from behind. Players should be taught to avoid head-first checking and head-first contact with the boards. They must wear properly fitting helmets.[19]

Gymnasts should be well supervised during practice. They and all others must avoid the use of the trampoline and minitrampoline, even at an elite level of competition.[6] In rugby, serious injury would be reduced by proper enforcement of the rules; conditioning exercises for the athletes' necks; proper matching of players by skill, size, and experience; and education of individuals about avoiding high-risk activities.[29] Better supervision may reduce injuries during horseback riding, as might quick-release stirrups. Many serious injuries result from being dragged along the ground with the foot caught in the stirrup.[4]

Finally, adults supervising activities for young people must be knowledgeable in the proper approach to handling an individual who may have a serious cervical spine injury. This educational task is formidable, given the millions of adults involved at all levels of physical education and competitive youth sports.

REFERENCES

1. Albright L. Head and neck injuries (revised). In: Committee on Sports Medicine, American Academy of Pediatrics. *Sports Medicine: Health Care for Young Athletes.* Evanston, IL: American Academy of Pediatrics; 1983:263-281
2. Gerberich SG, Priest JD, Boen JR, Straub CP, Maxwell RE. Concussion incidences and severity in secondary school varsity football players. *Am J Public Health.* 1983;73:1370-1375
3. Mueller FO, Blyth CS. Fatalities from head and cervical spine injuries occurring in tackle football: 40 years' experience. *Clin Sports Med.* 1987;6:185-196
4. Bruce DA, Schut L, Sutton LN. Brain and cervical spine injuries occurring during organized sports activities in children and adolescents. *Clin Sports Med.* 1982;1:495-514
5. Torg JS. Problems and prevention. In: Torg JS, ed. *Athletic Injuries to the Head, Neck, and Face.* Philadelphia, PA: Lea and Febiger; 1982:3-13
6. Clarke KS. An epidemiologic view. In: Torg JS, ed. *Athletic Injuries to the Head, Neck, and Face.* Philadelphia, PA: Lea and Febiger; 1982:15-25
7. Lehman LB. Nervous system sports-related injuries. *Am J Sports Med.* 1987;15:494-499
8. Rosman NP, Herskowitz J. Trauma to the brain and spinal cord. In: Swaiman KF, Wright FS, eds. *The Practice of Pediatric Neurology.* St. Louis, MO: CV Mosby Co; 1982:966-968
9. Yarnell PR, Lynch S. The "ding": amnesic states in football trauma. *Neurology.* 1973;23:196-197
10. Cantu RC. Guidelines for return to contact sports after a cerebral concussion. *Phys Sportsmed.* 1986;14:75-83
11. Bruce DA, Alavi A, Bilaniuk L, Dolinskas C, Obrist W, Uzzell B. Diffuse cerebral swelling following head injuries in children: the syndrome of "malignant brain edema." *J Neurosurg.* 1981;54:170-178
12. Bennett DR, Fuenning SI, Sullivan G, Weber J. Migraine precipitated by head trauma in athletes. *Am J Sports Med.* 1980;8:202-205
13. Haas DC, Pineda GS, Lourie H. Juvenile head trauma syndromes and their relationship to migraine. *Arch Neurol.* 1975;32:727-730
14. Vegso JJ, Lehman RC. Field evaluation and management of head and neck injuries. *Clin Sports Med.* 1987;6:1-15
15. Saunders RL, Harbaugh RE. The second impact syndrome in catastrophic contact-sports head trauma. *JAMA.* 1984;252:538-539
16. Gronwall D, Wrightson P. Delayed recovery of intellectual function after mild head injury. *Lancet.* 1974;2:605-609

17. Wilberger JE. Minor head trauma in athletes. *Neurotrauma Medical Report*. 1988;2:1,4
18. Torg JS, Vegso JJ, Sennett B. The National Football Head and Neck Injury Registry: 14-year report on cervical quadriplegia (1971-1984). *Clin Sports Med*. 1987;6:61-72
19. Tater CH. Neck injuries in ice hockey: a recent, unsolved problem with many contributing factors. *Clin Sports Med*. 1987;6:101-114
20. Selbst SM, Alexander D, Ruddy R. Bicycle-related injuries. *Am J Dis Child*. 1987;141:140-144
21. Shields CL Jr, Fox JM, Stauffer ES. Cervical cord injuries in sports. *Phys Sportsmed*. 1978;6(9):71-76
22. Torg JS, Wiesel SW, Rothman RH. Diagnosis and management of cervical spine injuries. In: Torg JS, ed. *Athletic Injuries to the Head, Neck, and Face*. Philadelphia, PA: Lea and Febiger; 1982:181-209
23. Torg JS. Management guidelines for athletic injury to the cervical spine. *Clin Sports Med*. 1987;6:53-60
24. Maroon JC. 'Burning hands' in football spinal cord injuries. *JAMA*. 1977;238:2049-2051
25. Pang D, Wilberger JE Jr. Spinal cord injury without radiographic abnormalities in children. *J Neurosurg*. 1982;57:114-129
26. Pavlov H. Radiographic evaluation of the cervical spine. In: Torg JS, ed. *Athletic Injuries to the Head, Neck, and Face*. Philadelphia, PA: Lea and Febiger; 1982:155-180
27. Torg JS, Pavlov H. Cervical spinal stenosis with cord neurapraxia and transient quadriplegia. *Clin Sports Med*. 1987;6:115-133
28. Jackson DW, Lohr FT. Cervical spine injuries. *Clin Sports Med*. 1986;5:373-386
29. Scher AT. Rugby injuries of the spine and spinal cord. *Clin Sports Med*. 1987;6:87-99

Table 32. Severity of Concussion*

Grade 1 (mild)	No loss of consciousness; anterograde amnesia <30 min
Grade 2 (moderate)	Loss of consciousness <5 min or anterograde amnesia of ≥30 min but <24 hr
Grade 3 (severe)	Loss of consciousness ≥5 min or anterograde amnesia ≥24 hr

*From Cantu RC. Guidelines for return to contact sports after a cerebral concussion. *Phys Sportsmed.* 1986;14(10):75-83 (Reprinted with permission.)

Table 33. Guidelines for Return to Play After Concussion*

	1st Concussion	2nd Concussion	3rd Concussion
Grade 1 (mild)	May return to play if asymptomatic.†	Return to play in 2 weeks if asymptomatic at that time for 1 week.	Terminate season; to play next season if asymptomatic.
Grade 2 (moderate)	Return to play after asymptomatic for 1 week.	Minimum of 1 month; may return to play then if asymptomatic for 1 week; consider terminating season.	Terminate season; may return to play next season if asymptomatic.
Grade 3 (severe)	Minimum of 1 month; may then return to play if asymptomatic for 1 week.	Terminate season; may return to play next season if asymptomatic.	

*From Cantu RC. Guidelines for return to contact sports after a cerebral concussion. *Phys Sportsmed.* 1986;14(10):75-83 (Reprinted with permission.)
†No headache; dizziness; or impaired orientation, concentration, or memory during rest or exertion.

CHAPTER 20

CHRONIC HEALTH PROBLEMS

Children with chronic illnesses (Table 34) have often been restricted from participating in formal and informal exercise programs, if not by the physiologic limitations imposed by their disease, then by physicians' instruction or parents' or coaches' fears of the dangers of exercise. Children in this situation can easily grow up viewing themselves as sickly or somehow incapable of participating in exercise. An important study[1] showed no relationship between objectively assessed exercise tolerance of children with tetralogy of Fallot and their families' predictions of their exercise tolerance. In fact, most children with chronic illnesses, like people in general, can benefit from exercise programs. In some cases, exercise testing can be of special diagnostic help, and, in some chronic health conditions, exercise programs can be of particular benefit, beyond the psychologic and fitness-related advantages that would accrue to any child (Table 34).

Respiratory Illnesses

Bronchial Asthma

Most children with asthma of any severity will exhibit exercise-induced asthma (EIA), also referred to as exercise-induced bronchospasm (EIB), under the appropriate inciting conditions. This near-universal outcome provides a major impediment to full participation by all asthmatic children in athletics and exercise programs and simultaneously provides a major tool for the clinician trying to diagnose atypical cases of reactive airways disease. The increase in airway resistance and the resulting fall in expiratory airflow *following* exercise have been recognized for centuries (Fig. 38). It is seen most reliably in the first 3 to 15 minutes after an 8- to 10-minute bout of exercise intense enough to cause an elevation of heart rate to 170 to 180 beats per minute. The asthmatic response is exaggerated by cold dry air, and can be blocked by warming and humidifying the inspired air. It has been suggested that EIA may even be independent of exercise itself and instead may be the result of airway cooling, since the response can be duplicated even at rest if the minute ventilation (especially with cold dry air) is large enough (Table 35).

The exclusion of asthmatic children and adolescents from exercise and sports programs because of the fear of inducing asthma attacks is especially unfortunate because most of these children can safely participate, and most EIA can be prevented (Table 36). Preexercise inhalation of beta agonist bronchodilators (eg, albuterol and metaproterenol) or cromolyn sodium will eliminate most postexercise problems in the asthmatic athlete and nonathlete. In some with relatively mild involvement, simple nonpharmacologic manipulations may even suffice. Wrapping a scarf around the face during jogging in cold weather will provide warmer and more humid air and thus a lower burden on the heat-exchanging capacity of the upper airway. Warm-up exercise to the point of wheezing, or even short of that point, may block subsequent EIA within the ensuing 1 to 2 hours (the so-called "refractory period"). Swimming may be encouraged instead of running as the sport of choice since it is the least likely of all sports to cause EIA, even for equal energy expenditure (most likely because of the high humidity of inspired air).

It is important to teach children with asthma, their parents, and coaches that asthma itself should not inhibit their participation in an active sports and exercise program. During each of the past six Olympic Games, gold medals in swimming have gone to athletes with asthma. In the 1984 Olympic Games, athletes with asthma won gold medals in basketball, cycling, rowing, swimming, track and field, and wrestling. More than 10% of the competitors on the U.S. team had EIA. For those few athletes competing on a national or international level, it is useful to know that cromolyn is now accepted by the International Olympic Committee, and albuterol and metaproterenol are also accepted if the athlete has a letter from a physician. Theophylline is legal but may result in unacceptably high caffeine levels because present drug testing technology may not be able to distinguish perfectly among the various xanthines.

Not all children with asthma need aspire to Olympic-level competition, but most should be able to participate at their own level in sports and exercise and may be interested to know that high-level competition is not out of the question simply because they have reactive airways. For the thousands of children with asthma who have avoided or have been excluded from normal play and school sports programs, it is important to emphasize that several studies have now shown conclusively that exercise programs—even running programs—are safe for children with asthma and that these programs can produce the same increases in fitness that they produce in nonasthmatic children.

Cystic Fibrosis (CF)

Patients with CF commonly suffer from exercise intolerance, generally related to the severity of their pulmonary involvement: the worse the airway obstruction, the lower the exercise tolerance. Some of the patients with the worst pulmonary function are at increased risk of developing arterial oxyhemoglobin desaturation during exercise. Most patients, even in the most severe group, will not desaturate; but since some will, it is advisable to perform an exercise test with ear oximetry or pulse oximetry in any patient whose forced expired volume in one second is less than 50% of predicted. This will make it possible to identify those patients whose saturation falls and to identify the exercise intensity (heart rate) at which desaturation occurs. The patients can then be advised to keep the intensity of their usual activities less than the critical level found in the laboratory. The role of supplemental oxygen during exercise is not yet clear (Table 37).

In addition to identifying patients who desaturate during exercise, there are several things to be learned from exercise testing in children and adolescents with CF. Fitness levels and maximal achievable power output can be monitored, as can heart rate and minute ventilation at submaximal workloads and rating of perceived exertion. For each of these variables, changes can be noted with natural disease progression or remission, or with medical intervention (including exercise conditioning intervention). With worse disease, fitness (VO_2max) and maximal workload will be lower; heart rate and ventilation at a given submaximal power will be higher. In addition, the exercise intensity will *seem* more difficult (have a higher rating of perceived exertion).

It is clear that most patients with CF, at all grades of pulmonary disease, can benefit from exercise conditioning programs with increased cardiopulmonary fitness and increased endurance of the ventilatory muscles. Results of studies differ as to whether pulmonary function improves or does not change and as to whether exercise can substitute for traditional therapies such as chest physical therapy and postural drainage in enhancing mucus clearance. Cystic fibrosis should not be allowed to prevent a child or adolescent from participating in exercise and sports programs.

Patients with CF lose more salt in their sweat than their healthy peers during single 90-minute bouts of exercise in the heat, and have significant decreases in serum chloride and sodium. They are able to adapt to repeated bouts of exercise in the heat, but they cannot correct the sweat defect. They continue to lose large amounts of sodium and chloride in sweat despite having improved metabolic responses to exercise and heat stress (lower heart rates and lower core body temperatures) after acclimation. Adolescents with CF who are given an unrestricted diet between daily sessions of exercise in the heat are able to correct serum sodium and chloride deficiencies on their own. Current recommendations, therefore, are to encourage CF patients who exercise in the heat to take in ample water and to have free access to the salt shaker at all times. Salt tablets are not necessary.

Diabetes Mellitus

Physical activity plays an important role in the management of young people with insulin-dependent diabetes. There are some special considerations concerning both single bouts and extended programs of increased activity for the youngster with diabetes. Glucose utilization increases with acute bouts of exercise, and insulin requirements decrease correspondingly unless glucose intake is appropriately increased. Without the proper adjustments, diabetic youngsters are at risk for developing hypoglycemia during exercise. The site of insulin injection influences serum glucose levels, with insulin injected into an exercising limb resulting in a fall in blood glucose. The same dose injected into a nonexercising limb, however, does not result in such a fall, probably because of the increased blood flow to the exercising limb compared to the one at rest.

Long-term exercise programs can improve fitness in the diabetic child, with the same benefits that accrue to other children. Avoiding obesity is of greater metabolic significance in young people with diabetes than in the normoglycemic population and is an important benefit of an exercise program. There is evidence that youngsters with diabetes who exercise regularly are able to maintain tighter diabetic control than their less active peers. The reasons for this are not clear, but there is also recent evidence that regular exercise may sensitize insulin receptors, resulting in chronic reduction of insulin requirements (Table 38).

Cardiac Disorders

Most children with congenital heart disease are able to participate in some forms of exercise quite safely. Many of these children will have low exercise tolerance, but this is caused at least in part by underactivity that has resulted from overprotection and caution on the part of parents, teachers, coaches, physicians, and often the children themselves.

Aortic Stenosis (AS)

For children and adolescents with this defect, exercise may actually be life-threatening. As many as 7% of patients with AS may die suddenly. Sudden death in AS usually occurs at rest, but may occur during exercise; therefore, these children should be evaluated by a pediatric cardiologist before they enter into an exercise program. Risk seems to be proportionate to the degree of stenosis and the resulting ventricular-arterial pressure gradient. Electrocardiogram (ECG) and blood pressure monitoring during a progressive exercise test may identify those patients who require catheterization and surgical repair. Most patients with pressure gradients of 20 mm Hg or less (which includes most patients with AS) can safely engage in even strenuous exercise.

Tetralogy of Fallot (TOF)

Children with TOF usually have low exercise tolerance before corrective surgery. Before surgery, patients generally restrict their own activity and need not be limited by prescription. After surgical correction, work tolerance approaches normal. This improvement is not seen after palliative surgery. After surgery, the main risk during exercise is dysrhythmia, which is not common but can be severe. An exercise test with an ECG may therefore be very useful in discovering which patients have exercise-associated dysrhythmia. Patients with no dysrhythmia may resume full activity after surgery.

Musculoskeletal and Neurologic Disorders

Muscular Dystrophy

Evidence of the effects of exercise on patients with muscular dystrophy is largely anecdotal. Some specialists feel that exercise hastens the progression of the disease; others feel that much of the rapid deterioration seen in adolescents once they become wheelchair bound can be attributed to inactivity. Exercise testing of any kind is extremely difficult in these patients (especially those with the Duchenne type) because they are likely to be too weak to pedal a cycle by the time they are old enough to be able to cooperate with testing instructions.

Scoliosis

Only very severe spinal deformity will directly influence exercise tolerance. Teen-agers with less severe curvature may also have diminished exercise tolerance because of inactivity. It is not clear from the medical literature whether patients with scoliosis can become more fit through conditioning, but there is nothing in their cardiorespiratory physiology that should interfere with attainment of fitness.

Pectus Excavatum

Exactly the same things apply in this form of chest wall deformity as apply in scoliosis, except that actual physiologic limits imposed by the defect itself are even rarer for pectus than for scoliosis. When there are limitations, they are likely to be subtle.

Epilepsy

Epilepsy that is well controlled by medication should not prevent a youngster from participating in a full exercise program. When seizures are not adequately controlled, activities during which a seizure would be dangerous to the patient (eg, scuba diving or bicycle racing) or to others (eg, riflery) should be prohibited. Exercise itself is not a cause of seizures, and there is no reason to prevent children whose epilepsy is in good control from playing collision sports.

Cerebral Palsy (CP)

Children and adolescents with CP often have greatly diminished exercise tolerance, largely because of their spasticity. A given external load requires much more effort because of the tremendous mechanical inefficiency (the energy that has gone into stumbling and righting oneself is not available to the task at hand).

Mental Retardation

Mentally retarded children often have low exercise tolerance because they are seldom given the opportunity to participate in exercise programs. Where such programs do exist for these children, the benefits –physical and emotional–are frequently great. The Special Olympics movement has helped bring the pleasures and some of the physical benefits of exercise and sports to this important segment of our population.

REFERENCE

1. Taylor MRH. *The response to exercise of children with congenital heart disease*. University of London; 1972. PHD Thesis. Cited in Godfrey S. *Exercise Testing in Children*. Philadelphia, PA: WB Saunders Co Ltd; 1974

Table 34. Chronic Health Problems

Respiratory
  Asthma
  Cystic fibrosis
Metabolic
  Diabetes mellitus
Cardiac
  Aortic stenosis
  Tetralogy of Fallot
Musculoskeletal
  Muscular dystrophy
  Scoliosis
  Pectus excavatum
Neurologic
  Epilepsy
  Cerebral palsy
  Mental retardation

Table 35. Features of Exercise-Induced Asthma

Typically *follows* exercise
Worse with cold air
Blocked with warm, humid air
Refractory period

Table 36. Prevention of Exercise-Induced Asthma

Nonpharmacologic
  scarf or facemask in cold weather
  sport choice (swimming vs running)
  warm-up exercise
Pharmacologic
  beta agonist inhalation (preceding exercise)
  cromolyn sodium inhalation (preceding exercise)

Table 37. Exercise in Cystic Fibrosis

Fitness and exercise tolerance:
   inversely related to severity of pulmonary disease

Oxyhemoglobin saturation during exercise:
   no change in most patients
   may fall in some patients with severe disease

Exercise in the heat:
   normal sweat volume
   excess electrolyte loss

Response to exercise programs:
   normal increase in fitness and work tolerance
   ? if improve pulmonary function

Table 38. Diabetes

Acute exercise
   ➡ blood glucose (especially if insulin injected in
     exercising muscle)

Exercise programs
   ⬆ fitness
   ⬇ obesity
   ⬇ insulin requirements

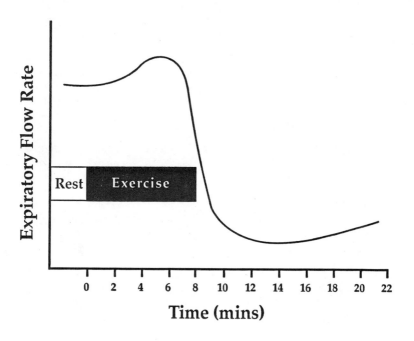

FIG. 38. Effect of Exercise on Expiratory Flow Rate.

Committee on Sports Medicine

Recommendations for Participation in Competitive Sports (RE8111)

The preparticipation physical examination is a frequent reason for adolescent visits to a pediatrician. The most commonly used list of disqualifying conditions, published by the American Medical Association, was last revised in 1976.[1] It has become increasingly obsolete because of changes in both safety equipment and society's attitudes toward the rights of athletes to compete despite a medical condition that may increase the risk of sustaining an injury or aggravating a

This statement has been approved by the Council on Child and Adolescent Health
The recommendations in this statement do not indicate an exclusive course of treatment or procedure to be followed. Variations, taking into account individual circumstances, may be appropriate.
PEDIATRICS (ISSN 0031 4005). Copyright © 1988 by the American Academy of Pediatrics.

preexisting medical condition. Most, if not all, sports are associated with some risk. The physician, the athlete, and the parents must weigh whether the advantages gained by participating in athletics are worth whatever risks are involved.

To assist practitioners in deciding whether athletes should be allowed to participate in particular sports, the American Academy of Pediatrics' Committee on Sports Medicine has compiled a list of recommendations. First, sport events were divided into groups depending on their degree of strenuousness and probability for collision (Figure). These groups of sports were then assessed in light of common medical and surgical conditions to determine whether participation would create a substantial risk of injury (Table).

Certain activities, such as skiing, are not inherently "contact sports." Yet, when competitors

| Contact/Collision | Limited Contact/Impact | Noncontact | | |
		Strenuous	Moderately Strenuous	Nonstrenuous
Boxing	Baseball	Aerobic dancing	Badminton	Archery
Field hockey	Basketball	Crew	Curling	Golf
Football	Bicycling	Fencing	Table tennis	Riflery
Ice hockey	Diving	Field		
Lacrosse	Field	Discus		
Martial arts	High jump	Javelin		
Rodeo	Pole vault	Shot put		
Soccer	Gymnastics	Running		
Wrestling	Horseback riding	Swimming		
	Skating	Tennis		
	Ice	Track		
	Roller	Weight lifting		
	Skiing			
	Cross-country			
	Downhill			
	Water			
	Softball			
	Squash, handball			
	Volleyball			

Figure. Classification of sports.

262 Appendices

TABLE. Recommendations for Participation in Competitive Sports

	Contact/ Collision	Limited Contact/Impact	Noncontact Strenuous	Noncontact Moderately Strenuous	Noncontact Nonstrenuous
Atlantoaxial instability	No	No	Yes*	Yes	Yes
* Swimming: no butterfly, breast stroke, or diving starts					
Acute illnesses	*	*	*	*	*
* Needs individual assessment, eg, contagiousness to others, risk of worsening illness					
Cardiovascular					
Carditis	No	No	No	No	No
Hypertension					
Mild	Yes	Yes	Yes	Yes	Yes
Moderate	*	*	*	*	*
Severe	*	*	*	*	*
Congenital heart disease	†	†	†	†	†
* Needs individual assessment.[2]					
† Patients with mild forms can be allowed a full range of physical activities; patients with moderate or severe forms, or who are postoperative, should be evaluated by a cardiologist before athletic participation.[2]					
Eyes					
Absence or loss of function of one eye	*	*	*	*	*
Detached retina	†	†	†	†	†
* Availability of American Society for Testing and Materials (ASTM)-approved eye guards may allow competitor to participate in most sports, but this must be judged on an individual basis.[3,4]					
† Consult ophthalmologist					
Inguinal hernia	Yes	Yes	Yes	Yes	Yes
Kidney: Absence of one	No	Yes	Yes	Yes	Yes
Liver: Enlarged	No	No	Yes	Yes	Yes
Musculoskeletal disorders	*	*	*	*	*
* Needs individual assessment					
Neurologic					
History of serious head or spine trauma, repeated concussions, or craniotomy	*	*	Yes	Yes	Yes
Convulsive disorder					
Well controlled	Yes	Yes	Yes	Yes	Yes
Poorly controlled	No	No	Yes†	Yes	Yes‡
* Needs individual assessment					
† No swimming or weight lifting					
‡ No archery or riflery					
Ovary: Absence of one	Yes	Yes	Yes	Yes	Yes
Respiratory					
Pulmonary insufficiency	*	*	*	*	Yes
Asthma	Yes	Yes	Yes	Yes	Yes
* May be allowed to compete if oxygenation remains satisfactory during a graded stress test					
Sickle cell trait	Yes	Yes	Yes	Yes	Yes
Skin: Boils, herpes, impetigo, scabies	*	*	Yes	Yes	Yes
* No gymnastics with mats, martial arts, wrestling, or contact sports until not contagious					
Spleen: Enlarged	No	No	No	Yes	Yes
Testicle: Absence or undescended	Yes*	Yes*	Yes	Yes	Yes
* Certain sports may require protective cup.[3]					

fall and collide with the ground, they are as much at risk as participants in the more traditional collision/contact sports. Hence, we have included such sports in a group called "limited contact/impact."

A list of all medical conditions that would disqualify athletes from participation would be nearly endless. Therefore, a concise table that can be consulted quickly and easily was thought to be most helpful. These, then, are the committee's recommendations for sports participation, to be referred to when the physician examines a young person with one of the listed conditions. Our recommendations should only be used as a guideline;

the physician's clinical judgment should remain the final arbiter in interpreting these recommendations for a specific patient.

COMMITTEE ON SPORTS MEDICINE, 1986–1988
Paul G. Dyment, MD, Chairman
Barry Goldberg, MD
Suzanne B. Haefele, MD
John J. Murray, MD
William L. Risser, MD
Michael A. Nelson, MD

Liaison Representatives
Oded Bar-Or, MD, Canadian Paediatric Society
Richard Malacrea, National Athletic Trainers Association

AAP Section Liaison
David M. Orenstein, MD, Section on Diseases of the Chest
Arthur M. Pappas, MD, Section on Orthopaedics

REFERENCES

1. American Medical Association: *Medical Evaluation of the Athlete: A Guide*, rev ed. Chicago, American Medical Association, 1976
2. Sixteenth Bethesda Conference: Cardiovascular abnormalities in the athlete: recommendations regarding eligibility for competition. *J Am Coll Cardiol* 1985;6:1186–1232
3. Dorsen PJ: Should athletes with one eye, kidney, or testicle play contact sports? *Phys Sportsmed* 1986;14:130–138
4. Vinger PF: The one-eyed athlete, editorial. *Phys Sportsmed* 1987;15:48–52

AMERICAN ACADEMY OF PEDIATRICS

Committee on Sports Medicine

Climatic Heat Stress and the Exercising Child
(RE2217)

Heat-induced illness is preventable. Physicians, teachers, coaches, and parents must be made aware of the potential hazards of high-intensity exercise in hot climates and of the measures needed to prevent heat-related illness in preadolescents.

Because of the following morphologic and functional differences, exercising children do not adapt to extremes of temperature as effectively as adults when exposed to a high-climatic heat stress.[1]

1. Children have a greater surface area-mass ratio than adults, which induces a greater heat transfer between the environment and the body.

2. Children produce more metabolic heat per mass unit than adults when walking or running.[2]

3. Sweating capacity is not as great in children as in adults.[3,4]

4. The capacity to convey heat by blood from the body core to the skin is reduced in the exercising child.[4,5]

The foregoing characteristics do not interfere with the ability of the exercising child to dissipate heat effectively in a neutral or mildly warm climate. However, when air temperature exceeds skin temperature, children have less tolerance to exercise than do adults. The greater the temperature gradient between the air and the skin, the greater the effect on the child.[4,6,7]

Upon transition to a warmer climate, any exercising individual must allow time for conditioning for heat (acclimatization). Intense and prolonged exercise undertaken before acclimatization may be detrimental to health and might even lead to fatal heat stroke.[8] Although children can acclimatize to exercise in the heat,[6,9] the rate of their acclimatization is slower than that of adults.[1] Therefore, a child will need more exposures to the new climate to sufficiently acclimatize.

Children frequently do not instinctively drink enough liquids to replenish fluid loss during prolonged exercise and may become gravely dehydrated.[10] A major consequence of dehydration is an excessive increase in body temperature during exercise. For a given level of dehydration, children are subject to a greater increase in core temperature than are adults.[10] Clinically, the dehydrated child is more prone to heat-related illness than the fully hydrated one.[11,12]

Children with the following conditions are at a potentially greater risk of heat stress: obesity, febrile state, cystic fibrosis, gastrointestinal infection, diabetes insipidus, diabetes mellitus, chronic heart failure, caloric malnutrition, anorexia nervosa, sweating insufficiency syndrome, and mental deficiency.

Based on the foregoing responses of children to exercise in hot climates, the Committee recommends:

1. The intensity of activities that last 30 minutes or more should be reduced whenever relative humidity and air temperature are above critical levels (zone 3 in Figure). Information concerning relative humidity may be obtained from a nearby US Weather Bureau or by use of a sling psychrometer (School Health Supplies, PO Box 409, 300 Lombard Rd, Addison, IL 60101; approximate cost $30) to compare dry bulb and wet bulb temperature levels.

2. At the beginning of a strenuous exercise program or after traveling to a warmer climate, the intensity and duration of exercise should be restrained initially and then gradually increased over a period of ten to 14 days to accomplish acclimatization to the effects of heat.

3. Prior to prolonged physical activity, the child should be fully hydrated. During the activity, periodic drinking (eg, 150 ml of cold tap water each 30 minutes for a child weighing 40 kg) should be enforced.

4. Clothing should be lightweight, limited to one layer of absorbent material in order to facilitate

PEDIATRICS (ISSN 0031 4005). Copyright © 1982 by the American Academy of Pediatrics.

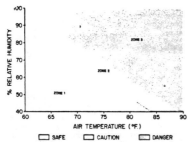

Figure. Weather guide for prevention of heat illness during prolonged strenuous exercise (Reproduced with permission from Mathews DK, Fox EL: *The Physiological Basis of Physical Education and Athletics*, ed 3. New York, CBC College Publishing (Holt, Rinehart & Winston, Inc, 1981.)

evaporation of sweat and expose as much skin as possible. Sweat-saturated garments should be replaced by dry ones. Rubberized sweat suits should never be used to produce loss of weight.

Proper health habits can be learned. The child athlete who may be exposed to a hot climate must be educated to observe the foregoing principles. Emphasis should be given to heat acclimatization, fluid intake, proper clothing, air temperature, and humidity.

COMMITTEE ON SPORTS MEDICINE (1979–1981)
Thomas E. Shaffer, MD, Chairman (1981–   )
Thomas G. Flynn, MD, Chairman (1978–1980)
Elizabeth Coryllos, MD
Paul G. Dyment, MD
John H. Kennell, MD
Eugene F. Luckstead, MD
Robert N. McLeod, Jr, MD
Nathan J. Smith, MD
William B. Strong, MD
Melvin L. Thornton, MD

Clemens W. Van Rooy, MD
John Murray, MD

Liaison Representatives:
Frederick W. Baker, MD, Canadian Paediatric
   Society
Lucille Burkett, American Alliance for Health,
   Physical Education and Recreation
Oded Bar-Or, MD, American College of
   Sports Medicine
Henry Levison, MD, Section on Diseases of
   the Chest
Richard Malacrea, National Athletic Trainers
   Association
James Moller, MD, Section on Cardiology

REFERENCES

1. Bar-Or O: Climate and the exercising child—A review. *Int J Sports Med* 1:53, 1980
2. Aastrand PO: *Experimental Studies of Physical Working Capacity in Relation to Sex and Age.* Copenhagen, Munksgaard, 1952
3. Haymes EM, McCormick RJ, Buskirk ER: Heat tolerance of exercising lean and obese prepubertal boys. *J Appl Physiol* 39: 457, 1975
4. Drinkwater BL, Kupprat IC, Denton JE, et al: Response of prepubertal girls and college women to work in the heat. *J Appl Physiol* 43:1046, 1977
5. Drinkwater BL, Horvath SM: Heat tolerance and aging. *Med Sci Sports* 11:49, 1979
6. Wagner JA, Robinson S, Tzankoff SP, et al: Heat tolerance and acclimatization to work in the heat in relation to age. *J Appl Physiol* 33:616, 1972
7. Haymes EM, Buskirk ER, Hodgson JL, et al: Heat tolerance of exercising lean and heavy prepubertal girls. *J Appl Physiol* 36:566, 1974
8. Fox EL, Mathews DK, Kaufman WS, et al: Effects of football equipment on thermal balance and energy cost during exercise. *Res Q Am Assoc Health Phys Educ Recreat* 37:332, 1966
9. Inbar O: *Acclimatization to Dry and Hot Environment in Young Adults and Children 8–10 Years Old*, dissertation, Columbia University, New York, 1978
10. Bar-or O, Dotan R, Inbar O, et al: Voluntary hypohydration in 10- to 12-year-old boys. *J Appl Physiol* 48:104, 1980
11. Danks DM, Webb DW, Allen J: Heat illness in infants and young children: A study of 47 cases. *Br Med J* 2:287, 1962
12. Taj-Eldin S, Falaki N: Heat illness in infants and small children in desert climates. *J Trop Med Hyg* 71:100, 1968
13. American College of Sports Medicine: Position statement on prevention of heat injuries during distance running. *Med Sci Sports* 7: 7, 1975

Committee on Sports Medicine

Anabolic Steroids and the Adolescent Athlete

(RE9135)

A major problem in both professional and elite amateur athletics is the misuse of anabolic steroids to increase muscle strength and/or muscle size. Their use is widespread among professional and college-level athletes, particularly in football players and weight lifters. These illicitly obtained drugs are readily available to athletes of almost any age; therefore, pediatricians must be concerned about the abuse of these drugs among their patients.[1]

In 1976, the International Olympic Committee on Drugs banned the use of anabolic steroids by competitors and placed severe sanctions on violators. A comprehensive review of the medical literature was undertaken in 1984 by the American College of Sports Medicine[2] and resulted in a position paper on anabolic steroid use in sports. In the paper, it was acknowledged that anabolic steroids can increase body weight (especially lean body weight) and, in combination with high-intensity weight training, can increase muscular strength in some highly conditioned athletes. It was also indicated that, although several controlled studies had been unable to demonstrate a strength advantage for those subjects taking the drugs, there were enough studies in which such an effect was shown to support the widespread belief among athletes that anabolic steroids are effective in increasing muscle power. The American College of Sports Medicine unequivocally condemned their use as performance-enhancing or "ergogenic" drugs.

Anabolic steroids (called "steroids" by athletes) are associated with a long list of potentially toxic effects.[2] Adverse effects on the liver include benign and malignant tumors, toxic hepatitis, and peliosis hepatitis, the latter a rare disturbance within the liver in which multiple blood lakes develop that can rupture spontaneously and cause severe hemor-

rhage. A recently recognized side effect is a decrease in serum high-density lipoprotein levels, which produces an atherogenic lipid profile with consequent possible increased risk of coronary artery disease.[3] Effects on the male reproductive system include oligospermia, azoospermia, decreased testicular size, and reduction of serum testosterone levels, all resulting from suppression of gonadotropic hormone production. Although serum lipid levels and testicular changes are reversible, concerns remain regarding their long-term effects. Psychologic changes attributed to steroids include mood swings, aggressive behavior, and changes in libido. Of particular concern to pediatricians is the premature closure of the epiphyses in prepubertal and early-pubertal youth. Virilization in women is a common side effect.

Pediatricians need to ask appropriate questions regarding the use of anabolic steroids and other ergogenic aids when performing preparticipation physical examinations. This is particularly important if the athlete competes in one of the power sports most associated with steroid misuse, such as football or weight lifting. Even if the athlete denies using anabolic steroids, anticipatory guidance concerning their side effects is appropriate for youths at risk.

The American Academy of Pediatrics agrees with the position statement of the American College of Sports Medicine in condemning the use of anabolic steroids by athletes. We deplore their use because of their known toxic side effects, because of our belief that taking ergogenic drugs is another form of cheating, and because competitors who enhance their athletic performance with anabolic steroids put the other competitors in the difficult position of either not taking them and conceding a perceived advantage to the abusing competitor or taking them as well and accepting the risks of untoward side effects. Young athletes should not be placed in the situation of having to make such a choice.

COMMITTEE ON SPORTS MEDICINE, 1986–1988
Paul G. Dyment, MD, Chairman
Barry Goldberg, MD

Suzanne B. Haefele, MD
William L. Risser, MD
Michael A. Nelson, MD
John J. Murray, MD

Liaison Representatives
Oded Bar-Or, MD, Canadian Paediatric
Society
Richard Malacrea, National Athletic
Trainers Association

AAP Section Liaisons
David M. Orenstein, MD, Section on
Diseases of the Chest
Arthur M. Pappas, MD, Section on
Orthopedics

REFERENCES

1. Dyment PG: The adolescent athlete and ergogenic aids. *J Adolesc Health Care* 1987;8:68-73
2. American College of Sports Medicine: Position statement on the use and abuse of anabolic/androgenic steroids in sports. *Med Sci Sports* 1987;19:534-539
3. Webb OL, Laskarzewski PM, Gleuck CJ: Severe depression of high-density lipoprotein cholesterol levels in weightlifters and body builders by self-administered exogenous testosterone and anabolic-androgenic steroids. *Metabolism* 1984;33:971-975

AMERICAN ACADEMY OF PEDIATRICS

**Committee on Accident and Poison Prevention and
Committee on Pediatric Aspects of Physical Fitness, Recreation,
and Sports**

Trampolines II   (RE2214)

In September 1977, the Academy published a statement calling for a ban on the use of trampolines in schools because of the high number of quadriplegic injuries caused by this apparatus.[1] A considerable amount of thought and action resulted. The Academy does not endorse trampoline use, but a revision of the Academy's position to allow for a trial period of limited and controlled use by schools seems appropriate. However, careful assessment of the incidence and severity of injury must continue during this trial period.

The trampoline is a potentially dangerous apparatus, and its use demands the following precautions:

1. The trampoline should not be a part of routine physical education classes.

2. The trampoline has no place in competitive sports.
3. The trampoline should *never* be used in home or recreational settings.
4. Highly trained personnel who have been instructed in all aspects of trampoline safety must be present, when the apparatus is used.
5. Maneuvers, especially the somersault, that have a high potential for serious injury should be attempted only by those qualified to become skilled performers.
6. The trampoline must be secured when not in use, and it must be well maintained.
7. Only schools or sports activities complying with the foregoing recommendations should have trampolines.

REFERENCE

1. Committee on Accident and Poison Prevention: *Trampolines*. Evanston, IL, American Academy of Pediatrics, September 1977

COMMITTEE ON ACCIDENT AND POISON
PREVENTION
H. James Holroyd, MD, Chairman
Lorne K. Garrettson, MD
Joseph Greensher, MD
Matilda S. McIntire, MD
Leonard S. Krassner, MD
Raymond Chi Wing Ng, MD
Avrin M. Overbach, MD
Barry H. Rumack, MD
Mark D. Widome, MD

Liaison Members
George D. Armstrong, National Clearinghouse for
  Poison Control Centers, Department of Health
  and Human Services
Diane Imhulse, National Safety Council
Andre l'Archeveque, MD, Canadian Paediatric So-
  ciety

H. Biemann Othersen, Jr, MD, Section on Surgery

COMMITTEE ON PEDIATRIC ASPECTS OF PHYSICAL
FITNESS, RECREATION, AND SPORTS
Thomas G. Flynn, MD, Chairman
John H. Kennell, MD
Robert N. McLeod, Jr, MD
Thomas E. Shaffer, MD
William B. Strong, MD
Melvin L. Thornton, MD
Clemens W. Van Rooy, MD

Liaison Members
Lucille Burkett, American Alliance for Health,
  Physical Education, Recreation and Dance
Fred W. Baker, MD, Canadian Paediatric Society
Richard Malacrea, National Athletic Trainers
  Association

A Self-Appraisal Checklist for Health Supervision in Scholastic Athletic Programs

Introduction

This checklist has been developed for use by school boards, superintendents, principals, athletic directors, coaches, trainers, and team physicians who are dedicated to providing excellent medical supervision for scholastic athletic programs. Sports medicine program staff may include one to several team physicians, school nurses, and athletic trainers.

The checklist consists of criteria for evaluation of the health aspects of scholastic athletic programs. Use of the checklist will help in evaluating the strengths, weaknesses, and adequacy of the sports medicine program and defining areas of inadequacies and needs for improvement. The checklist is designed to be a permanent reference source in each school. Evaluations should be performed annually to insure sound medical supervision of school sports to provide for the safety and protection of athletes.

The checklist is organized into six major categories which represent essential aspects of medical supervision of all scholastic athletics. While there are differences in various components of medical supervision between schools, the categories should be represented to some degree in each school. The checklist, therefore, can be useful to personnel in surveying and assessing its existing program and, in time, comparing it to a quality program exemplified by the checklist items.

How To Use This Checklist

The Self-Appraisal Checklist for Health Supervision in Scholastic Athletic Programs contains 64 items. Each item represents a criterion against which a sports medicine program can be judged. Evaluative criteria are presented in the form of statements which describe attributes of health supervision of athletes. Each statement sets forth a condition deemed highly desirable for an exemplary program. The evaluator should read carefully each statement and determine as objectively as possible the extent to which the statement describes the local program. This appraisal should be recorded by circling:

4, if the evaluator determines that the statement *always* describes the program

3, if the evaluator determines that the statement *sometimes* decribes the program

2, if the evaluator is *uncertain*

1, if the evaluator determines that the statement *seldom* decribes the program

0, if the evaluator determines that the statement *never* decribes the program

A 4 rating suggests that the stated attribute of the sports medicine program is very satisfactory; a 3 rating signifies satisfactory, and a 2 rating may identify a factor in the program that is borderline between satisfactory and unsatisfactory. A 1 rating suggests need for improvement and a 0 indicates that the attribute is missing in the program.

A *possible score* is given for each category, based upon a 4 rating for each statement. The *actual score* is the total of the ratings given by the evaluator. When the checklist has been completed, needed improvements in the program may be identified on the basis of discrepancies between actual and possible scores.

I. Philosophy and Principles

Possible Score — 36 points   Actual Score — _____ points

Circle appropriate response as related to your school
4 = Always
3 = Sometimes
2 = Uncertain
1 = Seldom
0 = Never

#	Statement	4	3	2	1	0
1.	There is a written statement expressing the philosophy, principles, and objectives of the athletic department.	4	3	2	1	0
2.	The stated philosophy expresses the need for physicians with interest and competence in sports medicine to be available to staff and athletes.	4	3	2	1	0
3.	The statement reflects the roles and responsibilities in the sports medicine program for coaches, parents, athletes, athletic trainers, and physicians.	4	3	2	1	0
4.	The school administration communicates this philosophy to all parents and athletes to help insure a clear understanding of policies.	4	3	2	1	0
5.	The statement is required reading for parents, coaches, and athletes.	4	3	2	1	0
6.	Sports medicine is regarded as an essential part of the total athletic program, not just as game or event coverage.	4	3	2	1	0
7.	The organization and function of the school's sports medicine program is under direction of a licensed physician.	4	3	2	1	0
8.	School personnel support recommendations of the sports medicine staff regarding treatment, rehabilitation, and the necessity to exclude certain athletes from participation for medical reasons.	4	3	2	1	0
9.	Parents' or guardians' consent for emergency medical treatment is on file with sports medicine personnel.	4	3	2	1	0

II. Organization and Administration

Possible Score — 48 points   Actual Score — ..... points

Circle appropriate response as related to your school
4 = Always
3 = Sometimes
2 = Uncertain
1 = Seldom
0 = Never

	Always	Sometimes	Uncertain	Seldom	Never
1. At least one athletic trainer, certified by the National Athletic Trainers' Association, is on the sports medicine staff.	4	3	2	1	0
2. The director of the sports medicine staff is responsible to the school administration for conducting a program to minimize sports injuries.	4	3	2	1	0
3. The athletic trainer is employed to treat and reduce the risks of sports injuries and is not involved in coaching.	4	3	2	1	0
4. A job description outlining duties and responsibilities of the sports medicine staff is available in writing.	4	3	2	1	0
5. There is an accessible file of individual health examination reports.	4	3	2	1	0
6. There is a method for maintaining records of weight, injuries, illnesses, and other pertinent information about the athletes.	4	3	2	1	0
7. There is a comprehensive insurance program for the medical care of injured athletes.	4	3	2	1	0
8. The director of the sports medicine program is a paid member of the staff.	4	3	2	1	0
9. The administration of the sports medicine program is delegated to a licensed physician whose responsibilities include planning, scheduling, organizing, supervising, and evaluating the total sports medicine program.	4	3	2	1	0
10. Equal opportunity is given to programs for both sexes in matters of policy, budget, use of facilities, equipment, scheduling, and the extent of participation.	4	3	2	1	0
11. A staffing pattern or chart is developed which specifies relationships among staff in the school sports program.	4	3	2	1	0
12. A systematic evaluation is used to maintain the effectiveness of the total program.	4	3	2	1	0

III. The Staff

Possible Score — 40 points   Actual Score — ___ points

	Circle appropriate response as related to your school
	4 = Always / 3 = Sometimes / 2 = Uncertain / 1 = Seldom / 0 = Never

1. The athletic director has professional preparation and experience necessary for planning and directing an interscholastic athletic program in a broad range of sports activities. — 4 3 2 1 0

2. The athletic director is involved in the selection of the athletic department staff, including sports medicine personnel. — 4 3 2 1 0

3. The athletic director encourages the sports medicine staff to attend professional meetings and educational programs in sports medicine. — 4 3 2 1 0

4. Coaches are knowledgeable in medical aspects of sports, including conditioning, care of the injured athlete, principles of rehabilitation and carry current certification in first aid and CPR. — 4 3 2 1 0

5. Coaches put the safety and health of the athlete as the highest priority. — 4 3 2 1 0

6. The sports medicine physicians are licensed to practice in the state. — 4 3 2 1 0

7. The physicians in the sports medicine program are involved in protecting the health of all athletes, are on call during practices, and attend all sports events that have high injury rates. — 4 3 2 1 0

8. The school has a National Athletic Trainers Association certified athletic trainer on the sports medicine staff. — 4 3 2 1 0

9. Aides to the certified staff personnel in the sports program have had training in first aid, basic life support, and CPR. — 4 3 2 1 0

10. The athletic director, coaches, athletic trainers and team physicians recognize that they are responsible as individuals, and also a team, for providing consistent, high standards in health care for young athletes. — 4 3 2 1 0

IV. Event Coverage

Possible Score — 40 points   Actual Score — _____ points

Circle appropriate response
as related to your school
4 = Always
3 = Sometimes
2 = Uncertain
1 = Seldom
0 = Never

#	Item	Always	Sometimes	Uncertain	Seldom	Never
1.	All coaches and sports medicine personnel are certified in CPR and trained in emergency managment of life-threatening injuries.	4	3	2	1	0
2.	Effective telephone access to a medical emergency unit is available.	4	3	2	1	0
3.	A suitable vehicle is available for immediate transportation of the injured athlete to a designated medical resource which has been altered.	4	3	2	1	0
4.	Competent adult supervision of the crowd is provided.	4	3	2	1	0
5.	The playing area is surveyed before each event to identify injury hazards on or near the field or court.	4	3	2	1	0
6.	A physician member of the sports medicine staff attends high risk sports events such as football, wrestling, hocky, and gymnastics, and events with a large spectator attendance.	4	3	2	1	0
7.	Emergency first aid supplies and equipment are *readily* available to all competing teams.	4	3	2	1	0
8.	Visiting teams have ready access to facilities for care of an injured athlete.	4	3	2	1	0
9.	Environmental conditions are monitored by sling psychrometer or other means during hot, humid weather and strenuous activity is modified as needed.	4	3	2	1	0
10.	Abundant supplies of drinking water and ice are available at all times.	4	3	2	1	0

V. Facilities and Equipment

Possible Score — 68 points   Actual Score — ___ points

Circle appropriate response
as related to your school
4 = Always
3 = Sometimes
2 = Uncertain
1 = Seldom
0 = Never

1. Adequate funds are allocated to the sports medicine program for:

a. expendable supplies	4	3	2	1	0
b. capital improvements	4	3	2	1	0
c. continuing education	4	3	2	1	0
d. repairs and maintenance	4	3	2	1	0

2. There is adequate space to handle the flow of routine care of the athletic population:

a. conditioning & reconditioning programs	4	3	2	1	0
b. prophylactic taping, wrapping, & padding	4	3	2	1	0
c. privacy for physical examinations	4	3	2	1	0
d. office space or station for record-keeping	4	3	2	1	0

3. There is an adequate supply of emergency equipment *readily* available, i.e.:

a. slings   f. stretcher
b. knee immobilizers g. spine board
c. crutches   h. sand bags
d. splints   i. equipment for maintaining an airway
e. cervical collar j. icepacks

	4	3	2	1	0
4. An adequate supply of first aid supplies is *readily* available.	4	3	2	1	0
5. There is an adequate and *readily* available communication system between the athletic participation areas and medical or para-medical assistance.	4	3	2	1	0
6. There is an established written transportation plan for the injured athlete in					
a. emergency situation	4	3	2	1	0
b. non-emergency situation	4	3	2	1	0
7. There are adequate provisions for heating or cooling body areas.	4	3	2	1	0
8. Sanitation and safety of players and staff are assured by written policies and proper facilities.	4	3	2	1	0
9. All electrical supply in the sports medicine area is controlled by ground fault interruptors at the outlet or control panel.	4	3	2	1	0
10. Adequate sports medicine facilities are available to all competing teams.	4	3	2	1	0

VI. Education

Possible Score — 24 points   Actual Score ——— points

Circle appropriate response
as related to your school
4 = Always
3 = Sometimes
2 = Uncertain
1 = Seldom
0 = Never

1. The sports medicine staff conducts educational sessions for all athletes. covering the following:

a. heat illness	4	3	2	1	0
b. nutrition	4	3	2	1	0
c. harmful effects of drugs, alcohol and tobacco	4	3	2	1	0
d. general hygiene for the athlete	4	3	2	1	0
e. rehabilitation after injury	4	3	2	1	0

2. The school makes available, for selected students, an elective course for athletic trainer aides.

	4	3	2	1	0

Summary of Scores

		Possible Score	Actual Score	%
Part I.	Philosophy and Principles	36		
Part II.	Organization and Administration	48		
Part III.	The Staff	40		
Part IV.	Facilities and Equipment	68		
Part V.	Event Coverage	40		
Part VI.	Education	24		
	Totals	256		

Committee on Sports Medicine

Participation in Boxing Among Children and Young Adults (RE2219)

The American Academy of Pediatrics opposes boxing in any sports program for children and young adults. Amateur boxing is potentially dangerous and yet youngsters are involved in boxing at ages 3 to 4 years. Approximately 15,000 boxers between ages 10 and 15 years are registered with the National Amateur Athletic Union (AAU) Junior Olympics boxing program.[1] There may be an even larger number of young boxers in community organizations. Impoverished youths view boxing as a means of financial gain with the potential of providing a new life. Unfortunately, for many, it is a means of improving their physical condition at the risk of slow progressive brain injury, with occasional or no financial rewards. Other sports offer the same conditioning opportunity with minimal or no risk of brain injury.

In contrast to professional boxing, amateur boxing is apparently for prestige, recognition, and the enjoyment of winning. Proponents of boxing suggest that it teaches self-defense and discipline, that it builds character and confidence, and that it is relatively safe. Opponents of boxing stress that the principal goal is to render the opponent senseless.

Ironically, protective headgear may actually increase brain injuries.[2] The degree of physical injury in boxing correlates with the physical strength and activity of the participants; the greatest risks exist when participants are obviously mismatched. The fatality rate in boxing is reported to be low.[3] However, the frequency of chronic brain damage is an increasing concern in the medical community.[1,4-6]

Recent studies[4-6] using computed tomography (CT) scanning have revealed brain injury in young boxers. Detection of such brain injury was previously missed by EEG, neurologic testing, and other standard prefight medical examination procedures. Studies[2,6-10] have shown that neuropathologic changes occur in human beings or animals knocked unconscious from a blunt blow to the head. "Accumulated destructive (brain) effects of repeated blows even when consciousness and posture are not lost are well known and accepted."[6]

It is unlikely that boxing will ever be abolished in the United States; therefore, it is crucial for pediatricians to become vigorous *opponents* of boxing as a sport for *any* child or young adult. Simple changes in rules and medical supervision, and increased awareness of the dangers of boxing are not enough. Our opposition to boxing should be expressed at the time of health maintenance or preparticipation examination; opposition should be expressed in public whenever the opportunity presents itself; and our opposition should be expressed as a printed recommendation in brochures available in pediatric waiting rooms. Children and young adults should be encouraged to participate in sports in which intentional head injury is not the primary objective of the sport.

COMMITTEE ON SPORTS MEDICINE, 1983–1984
Thomas E. Shaffer, MD, Chairman
Paul G. Dyment, MD
Eugene F. Luckstead, MD
John J. Murray, MD
Nathan J. Smith, MD

Liaison Representatives
James H. Moller, MD
    Section on Cardiology
David M. Orenstein, MD
    Section on Diseases of the Chest
Arthur M. Pappas, MD
    Section on Orthopaedics
Frederick W. Baker, MD
    Canadian Paediatric Society
Richard Malacrea
    National Athletic Trainers Association

This statement has been approved by the Council on Child and Adolescent Health.
PEDIATRICS (ISSN 0031 4005). Copyright © 1984 by the American Academy of Pediatrics.

REFERENCES

1. American Medical Association Council on Scientific Affairs Report: Brain injury in boxing. *JAMA* 1983;249:254–257

2. Timperley WR: Banning boxing, letter. *Br Med J* 1982;285:289
3. Some high risk sports, editorial. *Sporting News*, Aug 16, 1960, p 14
4. Casson IR, Sham R, Campbell EA, et al: Neurological and CT evaluation of "knocked out" boxers. *J Neurol Neurosurg Psychiatry* 1982;45:170-174
5. Kaste M, Kuurne T, Vilkki J, et al: Is chronic brain damage in boxing a hazard of the past? *Lancet* 1982;2:1186-1188
6. Ross RJ, Cole M, Thompson JS, et al: Boxers: Computed tomography, EEG and neurological evaluation. *JAMA* 1983;249:211-213
7. Lundberg GD: Boxing should be banned in civilized countries, editorial. *JAMA* 1983;249:250
8. Van Allen MW: The deadly degrading sport, editorial. *JAMA* 1983;249:250-251
9. Gronwall D, Wrightson P: Cumulative effects of concussion, letter. *Lancet* 1979;2:995-997
10. Corsellis JAN, Bruton CJ, Freeman-Browne D: The aftermath of boxing. *Psychol Med* 1973;3:270-303

SPORTS PARTICIPATION HEALTH RECORD

This evaluation is only to determine readiness for sports participation. It should not be used as a substitute for regular health maintenance examinations.

NAME _____ AGE _____ (YRS) GRADE _____ DATE _____

ADDRESS _____ PHONE _____

SPORTS _____

The Health History (Part A) and Physical Examination (Part C) sections must both be completed, at least every 24 months, before sports participation. The Interim Health History section (Part B) needs to be completed at least annually.

PART A — HEALTH HISTORY:
To be completed by athlete and parent

	YES	NO
1. Have you ever had an illness that:		
a. required you to stay in the hospital?	___	___
b. lasted longer than a week?	___	___
c. caused you to miss 3 days of practice or a competition?	___	___
d. is related to allergies? (ie, hay fever, hives, asthma, insect stings)	___	___
e. required an operation?	___	___
f. is chronic? (ie, asthma, diabetes, etc)	___	___
2. Have you ever had an injury that:		
a. required you to go to an emergency room or see a doctor?	___	___
b. required you to stay in the hospital?	___	___
c. required x-rays?	___	___
d. caused you to miss 3 days of practice or a competition?	___	___
e. required an operation?	___	___
3. Do you take any medication or pills?	___	___
4. Have any members of your family under age 50 had a heart attack, heart problem, or died unexpectedly?	___	___
5. Have you ever:		
a. been dizzy or passed out during or after exercise?	___	___
b. been unconscious or had a concussion?	___	___
6. Are you unable to run 1/2 mile (2 times around the track) without stopping?	___	___
7. Do you:		
a. wear glasses or contacts?	___	___
b. wear dental bridges, plates, or braces?	___	___
8. Have you ever had a heart murmur, high blood pressure, or a heart abnormality?	___	___
9. Do you have any allergies to any medicine?	___	___
10. Are you missing a kidney?	___	___

11. When was your last tetanus booster? _____

12. For Women
a. At what age did you experience your first menstrual period? _____
b. In the last year, what is the longest time you have gone between periods? _____

EXPLAIN ANY "YES" ANSWERS _____
_____
_____

I hereby state that, to the best of my knowledge, my answers to the above questions are correct.

Date _____

Signature of athlete _____

Signature of parent _____

PART B — INTERIM HEALTH HISTORY:
This form should be used during the interval between preparticipation evaluations. Positive responses should prompt a medical evaluation.

1. Over the next 12 months, I wish to participate in the following sports:
a. _____
b. _____
c. _____
d. _____

2. Have you missed more than 3 consecutive days of participation in usual activities because of an injury this past year?
Yes _____ No _____
If yes, please indicate:
a. Site of injury _____
b. Type of injury _____

3. Have you missed more than 5 consecutive days of participation in usual activities because of an illness, or have you had a medical illness diagnosed that has not been resolved in this past year?
Yes _____ No _____
If yes, please indicate:
a. Type of illness _____

4. Have you had a seizure, concussion or been unconscious for any reason in the last year?
Yes _____ No _____

5. Have you had surgery or been hospitalized in this past year?

Yes _____ No _____

If yes, please indicate:

a. Reason for hospitalization _____

b. Type of surgery _____

6. List all medications you are presently taking and what condition the medication is for.

a. _____

b. _____

c. _____

7. Are you worried about any problem or condition at this time?

Yes _____ No _____

If yes, please explain: _____

_____

_____

I hereby state that, to the best of my knowledge, my answers to the
above questions are correct.

Date _____

Signature of athlete _____

Signature of parent _____

Part C – PHYSICAL EXAMINATION RECORD

NAME _____ DATE _____ AGE _____ BIRTHDATE _____

Height _____ Vision: R _____ / _____ , corrected _____ , uncorrected _____

Weight _____ L _____ / _____ , corrected _____ , uncorrected _____

Pulse _____ Blood Pressure _____ Percent Body Fat (optional) _____

	Normal	Abnormal Findings	Initials
1. Eyes			
2. Ears, Nose, Throat			
3. Mouth & Teeth			
4. Neck			
5. Cardiovascular			
6. Chest and Lungs			
7. Abdomen			
8. Skin			
9. Genitalia - Hernia (male)			
10. Musculoskeletal: ROM, strength, etc.			
a. neck			
b. spine			

	1.	2.	3.	4.	5.
c. shoulders					
d. arms/hands					
e. hips					
f. thighs					
g. knees					
h. ankles					
i. feet					
11. Neuromuscular					
12. Physical Maturity (Tanner Stage)					

Comments re: Abnormal Findings: _____

_____

_____

PARTICIPATION RECOMMENDATIONS:

1. No participation in: _____

2. Limited participation in: _____

3. Requires: _____

4. Full participation in: _____

Physician Signature _____

Telephone Number _____ Address _____

American Academy of Pediatrics

Committee on Sports Medicine

Strength Training, Weight and Power Lifting, and Body Building by Children and Adolescents (RE9196)

Some children and many adolescents use weights to increase strength or enlarge muscles. A smaller number compete in the sports of weight lifting, power lifting, and body building.

DEFINITIONS

Free weights are dumbbells and barbells that are used without the external support of a machine.

Major lifts are lifts used in the sports of weight and power lifting. Also used are the power clean and the incline and overhead presses. These lifts involve the use of free weights lifted through the extremes of joint motion in a ballistic rather than a controlled fashion. They have significant potential to cause injury.[1-3] In the clean and jerk, the athlete lifts the barbell in a two-step movement from the floor to the chest and then over the head; the snatch involves the same movement of the barbell performed without interruption with a different technique. The power clean requires raising the barbell from the floor to the shoulders in a two-part maneuver. The dead lift is accomplished by raising the barbell from the floor by straightening the flexed knees. In the squat lift, the athlete holds the barbell behind the head on the shoulders, squats until the thighs are parallel with the floor, and then straightens the legs. In the bench press, the athlete lies supine on a bench, holds the barbell over the chest with the arms extended, lowers the weight to the chest, and then raises it again. The incline press is similar, except that the bench is at a 30° angle. In the overhead press, the lifter stands and raises the barbell from in front of the chest to over the head by extending the arms.

This statement has been approved by the Council on Child and Adolescent Health.

The recommendations in this statement do not indicate an exclusive course of treatment or procedure to be followed. Variations, taking into account individual circumstances, may be appropriate.

PEDIATRICS (ISSN 0031 4005). Copyright © 1990 by the American Academy of Pediatrics.

Strength training ("weight training," "resistance training") is the use of a variety of methods, including exercises with free weights and weight machines, to increase muscular strength, and/or power for sports participation or fitness enhancement.

Weight lifting and power lifting are competitive sports in which an athlete attempts to lift a maximal amount of free weight in specific lifts. In weight lifting, the lifts performed are the clean and jerk and the snatch. In power lifting, they are the squat lift, dead lift, and bench press.

Body building is a competitive sport in which the participant uses several resistance training methods, including free weights, to develop muscle size, symmetry, and definition.

STRENGTH TRAINING IN THE PREPUBESCENT ATHLETE

Recent research has shown that short-term programs in which prepubescent athletes are trained and supervised by knowledgeable adults can increase strength without significant injury risk.[4-6] These studies did not evaluate the relationship between improved strength, injury prevention, or enhanced athletic performance. No data exist defining risks of injury in less well-organized programs.

STRENGTH TRAINING IN THE PUBESCENT AND POSTPUBESCENT ATHLETE

Interscholastic athletic programs in secondary schools are increasingly emphasizing strength training as a conditioning method for participants in male and female sports. The major lifts are often used.

Although the incidence is unknown, strength training in adolescence occasionally produces significant musculoskeletal injury, eg, epiphyseal fractures, ruptured intervertebral disks, and low back bony disruptions, especially during use of the major lifts.[1-3] Safety requires careful planning of several aspects of a program. This includes devising a program for the intensity, duration, frequency, and rate of progression of weight use, as well as selection of sport-specific exercises appropriate for the physical maturity of the individual. Proper supervision should be provided during training sessions.[7-9]

WEIGHT LIFTING, POWER LIFTING, AND BODY BUILDING

More than 600 teenagers are registered with the United States Weight Lifting Federation, and more than 3000 with the United States Power Lifting Federation. The limited available data indicate that these sports have a significant risk of injury. Brown and Kimball[3] determined that 71 adolescent power lifters with a mean age of 16 years and a mean duration of 17 months participation sustained 98 musculoskeletal injuries, causing discontinuance of training for a total of 1126 days. Body building, with at least 8500 adolescent participants, uses some of the same exercises and presumably is associated with the same risks.

LIFTING MAXIMAL AMOUNTS OF WEIGHT

Because very little data are available on the relative rate of injury at different ages, controversy exists concerning when young athletes should be allowed to lift maximal amounts of weight. The United States Weight and Power Lifting Federations recommend the age of 14 years. Other experts suggest an older age, for example 16 years.[7] Given the widely varying tempo of pubertal development among adolescents, a more appropriate guideline is one based on physical maturation. If male and female athletes have reached Tanner stage 5 in the development of their secondary sexual characteristics, they will have passed their period of maximal velocity of height growth,[10,11] during which the epiphyses appear to be especially vulnerable to injury.[12] This level of developmental maturity is reached at a mean age of approximately 15 years in both sexes, with much individual variation.[10,11]

TRAINING FOR COACHES

It is essential that coaches have training in supervising strength training programs. Adequate instruction may be obtained in collegiate or graduate school programs or from continuing education courses offered by college strength training instructors. A convenient training program of high quality is offered by the National Strength and Conditioning Association,[*] with home study of written materials and videotapes followed by a certification examination.

RECOMMENDATIONS

The American Academy of Pediatrics recommends:

1. Strength training programs for prepubescent, pubescent, and postpubescent athletes should be permitted only if conducted by well-trained adults. The adults should be qualified to plan programs appropriate to the athlete's stage of maturation, which should be assessed objectively by medical personnel.

2. Unless good data become available that demonstrate safety, children and adolescents should avoid the practice of weight lifting, power lifting, and body building, as well as the repetitive use of maximal amounts of weight in strength training programs, until they have reached Tanner stage 5 level of developmental maturity.

COMMITTEE ON SPORTS MEDICINE, 1989–1990
Michael A. Nelson, MD, Chairman
Barry Goldberg, MD
Sally S. Harris, MD
Gregory L. Landry, MD
William L. Risser, MD

Liaison Representatives
Oded Bar-Or, MD, Canadian Paediatric
    Society
Richard Malacrea, National Athletic
    Trainers Association
Roswell Merrick, National Association
    for Sport and Physical Education

AAP Section Liaison
David M. Orenstein, MD, Section on
    Diseases of the Chest
Arthur M. Pappas, MD, Section on
    Orthopaedics

REFERENCES

1. Brady TA, Cahill BR, Bodnar LM. Weight training-related injuries in the high school athlete. Am J Sports Med. 1982;10:1 5

2. Gumbs VL, Segal D, Halligan JB, et al. Bilateral distal radius and ulnar fractures in adolescent weight lifters. Am J Sports Med. 1982;10:375-379

3. Brown EW, Kimball RG. Medical history associated with adolescent powerlifting. Pediatrics. 1983;72:636-644

4. Sewal L, Micheli LJ. Strength training for children. J Pediatr Orthop. 1986;6:143-146

5. Rians CB, Weltman A, Cahill BR, et al. Strength training for prepubescent males: is it safe? Am J Sports Med. 1987;15:483 489

6. Servedio FJ, Bartels RL, Hamlin RL, et al. The effects of weight training using Olympic lifts on various physiological variables in pre-pubescent boys. Med Sci Sports Exerc. 1985;17:288

7. Fleck SJ, Kraemer WJ. Designing Resistance Training Pro-

grams. Champaign, IL: Human Kinetics Books; 1987
8. *How to Build a Strength and Conditioning Program in Your High School*. National Strength and Conditioning Association. PO Box 81410, Lincoln, NE 68501. Tel. 402-472-3000
9. Cahill BR. ed. Proceedings of the Conference on Strength Training in the Prepubescent; 1988; Chicago. American Orthopaedic Society for Sports Medicine, 70 West Hubbard St, Suite 202, Chicago, IL 60610
10. Marshall WA, Tanner JM. Variations in the pattern of pubertal changes in girls. *Arch Dis Child.* 1969;44:291–303
11. Marshall WA, Tanner JM. Variations in the pattern of pubertal changes in boys. *Arch Dis Child.* 1970;45:13–23
12. Smith NJ, Stanitski CL. *Sports Medicine.* Philadelphia, PA: WB Saunders Co; 1987:33

Committee on Sports Medicine

Risks in Distance Running for Children (RE9192)

In recent years, there has been a surge in the participation of children in distance running. It is not unusual for an aspiring prepubescent athlete to run 10 to 15 miles daily and to participate in distance races, including marathons (26.2 miles).

Although running is a natural activity that can maintain and improve aerobic fitness, racing and particularly training for long distances have their risks. Distance running may induce musculoskeletal, endocrine, hematologic, thermoregulatory, and psychosocial damage. Most reports on such potential damage have not been evaluated with proper epidemiologic scrutiny. It is unknown whether the risk is greater for children than for adults. Nevertheless, the American Academy of Pediatrics wishes to alert the physician to the presence of such risks. Even without established guidelines and extensive documentation, physicians can give children, parents, and coaches advice that fosters healthy physical and psychosocial growth.

The most common musculoskeletal problems in the young runner are overuse injuries (ie, those that result from a mechanical stress repeated during a long period). These include epiphyseal plate injuries, stress fractures, patellofemoral syndrome, and chronic tendonitis.[1-4] The incidence of such injuries seems to be related to the total distance covered in training and competition.[4] Such overuse injuries may lead to a chronic disability (eg, chronic arthritis and growth deformity). Therefore, early medical intervention is important.

Female distance runners often experience delayed menarche.[5] Its etiology and relevance to health have yet to be established. In most cases, menarche will occur several months after cessation or reduction in volume of training. When a female athlete displays a delayed menarche, a medical etiology should be considered—rather than assuming causation by exercise.[6]

Although studies have not been performed in prepubertal children, iron depletion, manifested by low serum ferritin concentration, even with a normal hemoglobin concentration, is not uncommon among adolescent runners of both sexes.[7] An iron-poor diet is probably a main contributor to this disorder. Hemolysis is an often-cited cause of iron loss in runners and is manifested by low serum haptoglobin levels.[8] One possible mechanism is repetitious foot strike (previously known as "march hemoglobinuria"). Hematuria and mild occult gastrointestinal bleeding have been observed and may contribute to iron depletion.

A child's ability to maintain thermal homeostasis during prolonged running is less efficient than that of an adult, particularly when the climate is very hot or very cold.[9] This deficiency may result in heat- or cold-related disorders, including heatstroke or hypothermia. Of particular concern is the dehydration that accompanies prolonged running, even if the child is given fluid *ad libitum*.[10] In addition, children take longer than adults to acclimatize to hot, humid climates, which further increases their risk for heat-related disorders.[9]

Psychologic and social problems for the child runner can result from spending long hours in training and setting unrealistic goals. This is similar to the effects of participation in other competitive sports, in which the child may be submitted to inappropriate pressures. A prepubertal child should be allowed to participate for the enjoyment of running, without fear of parental or peer rejection or pressure.

Total mileage (and number of hours) covered by the child during training rather than the distance run on the day of competition may entail the greatest risk to the child's well-being and health. Therefore, suggestions cannot be made for specific maximal racing distances for children. It is important to recognize, however, that heat-related disorders are particularly pronounced in races that exceed 30 minutes in duration.

Until further data are available concerning the

This statement has been approved by the Council on Child and Adolescent Health.
PEDIATRICS (ISSN 0031 4005). Copyright © 1990 by the American Academy of Pediatrics.

relative risk of endurance running at different ages, the American Academy of Pediatrics recommends that, if children enjoy the activity and are asymptomatic, there is no reason to preclude them from training for and participating in such events. The risks discussed in this statement should be considered by pediatricians when counseling families about the advisability of their children participating in distance running.

COMMITTEE ON SPORTS MEDICINE, 1989–1990
Michael A. Nelson, MD, Chairman
Barry Goldberg, MD
Sally S. Harris, MD
Gregory L. Landry, MD
William L. Risser, MD

Liaison Representatives
Oded Bar-Or, MD, Canadian Paediatric Society
Richard Malacrea, National Athletic Trainers Association
Roswell Merrick, National Association for Sport and Physical Education

AAP Section Liaison
David M. Orenstein, MD, Section on Diseases of the Chest

Arthur M. Pappas, MD, Section on Orthopaedics

REFERENCES

1. Caine DJ, Koenraad JL. Growth plate injury: a threat to young distance runners? *Physician Sportsmed.* 1984;12:118–124
2. Chandy TA, Grana WA. Secondary school athletic injury in boys and girls: a three-year comparison. *Physician Sportsmed.* 1985;13:106–111
3. Micheli LJ, Santopietro F, Gerbino P, Growe MD. Etiologic assessment of overuse stress fractures in athletics. *Nova Scotia Med Bull.* April/June 1980:43–47
4. Orava S, Saarela J. Exertion injuries to young athletes: a follow-up research of orthopaedic problems of young track and field athletes. *Am J Sports Med.* 1978;6:68–74
5. Malina RM. Menarche in athletes: a synthesis and hypothesis. *Ann Hum Biol.* 1983;10:1–24
6. Shangold MM. Menstruation. In: Shangold MM, Mirkin G, eds. *Women and Exercise.* Philadelphia, PA: F.A. Davies; 1988:129–144
7. Nickerson HJ, Tripp AD. Iron deficiency in adolescent cross-country runners. *Physician Sportsmed.* 1983;11:60–66
8. Rowland TW. Iron deficiency and supplementation in the young endurance athlete. In: Bar-Or O, ed. *Advances in Pediatric Sport Sciences.* Champaign, IL: Human Kinetics; 1989;3:169–190
9. Bar-Or O. *Pediatric Sports Medicine for the Practitioner.* New York, NY: Springer Verlag; 1983
10. Bar-Or O, Dotan R, Inbar O, Rotshtein A, Zonder H. Voluntary hypohydration in 10- to 12-year-old boys. *J Appl Physiol.* 1980;48:104–108

Committee on Sports Medicine

Knee Brace Use by Athletes (RE9175)

The knee is the most frequently injured joint during athletic events, and the medial collateral ligament is one of the most frequently injured ligamentous structures of the knee. The medial collateral ligament is a prime stabilizer of the medial side of the knee. The most frequent cause of injury to this ligament is a blow from the lateral side of the knee or thigh with or without a rotatory force, which causes a valgus stress. In the growing child, similar forces to the lateral side of the knee may result in a femoral fracture due to displacement of the distal epiphysis.

It has become a goal of sports medicine enthusiasts to decrease the number of knee injuries and, specifically, the medial knee injury. The most readily apparent method to protect the knee is to provide additional external support. The lateral unidirectional articulated knee brace, strapped to the thigh and the calf, was developed in an attempt to reduce knee injuries. These lateral knee-stabilizing braces, the so-called "prophylactic knee braces," have become widely used by football players at all levels of skill. A number of early reports provided mixed conclusions as to the value of these braces.[1] Two recent comprehensive studies both concluded that so-called preventive braces are not preventive and may, in fact, be harmful.[2,3]

Based on current evidence, the American Academy of Pediatrics recommends that lateral unidirectional knee braces not be considered standard equipment for football players because of lack of efficacy and the potential of actually causing harm.

COMMITTEE ON SPORTS MEDICINE, 1989–1990
Michael A. Nelson, MD, Chairman
Barry Goldberg, MD
Sally S. Harris, MD
Gregory L. Landry, MD
William L. Risser, MD

Liaison Representatives
Oded Bar-Or, MD, Canadian Paediatric Society
Richard Malacrea, National Athletic Trainers Association
Roswell Merrick, National Association for Sport and Physical Education

AAP Section Liaison
David M. Orenstein, MD, Section on Diseases of the Chest
Arthur M. Pappas, MD, Section on Orthopaedics

REFERENCES

1. France EP, Paulos LE, Jayaraman G, Rosenberg TD. Biomechanics of lateral knee bracing, II: impact response of the braced knee. Am J Sports Med. 1987;15:430-438
2. Teitz CC, Hermanson BK, Kronmal RA, et al. Evaluation of the use of braces to prevent injury to the knee in collegiate football players. J Bone Joint Surg Am. 1987;69:2-9
3. Grace TG, Skipper BJ, Newberry JC, et al. Prophylactic knee braces and injury to the lower extremity. J Bone Joint Surg Am. 1988;70:422-427

AMERICAN ACADEMY OF PEDIATRICS

Committee on Sports Medicine and Committee on School Health

Organized Athletics for Preadolescent Children

(RE9165)

Each year in the United States, millions of preadolescent children participate in organized athletics. Some organized athletic programs are community based; others are school sponsored, either as extracurricula programs or as part of physical education classes. Most coaches in community-based programs are volunteers who have no formal training or expertise in coaching. The credentials and training of grade school coaches are highly variable. Therefore, many US preadolescents are involved in athletics without the benefit of specific program goals aimed at ensuring the most beneficial physical, psychologic, and recreational outcomes.

Coaches, officials, parents, and program designers all play critical roles in shaping the child's early athletic experience and the child's self-esteem. The goals of the program and the behavior of all of the adults involved should focus upon assisting the child to develop: (1) an enjoyment of sports and fitness that will be sustained through adulthood, (2) physical fitness,[1] (3) basic motor skills, (4) a positive self-image, (5) a balanced perspective on sports in relation to the child's school and community life, and (6) a commitment to the values of teamwork, fair play, and sportsmanship. In addition, efforts must be made to make the sport as safe as possible.

Enjoyment of sports and fitness in childhood will increase the likelihood of a child pursuing these activities through adulthood. Children should be allowed to try a variety of sports and to choose sports that appeal to them. If children require more than gentle encouragement, then they are not ready for involvement. Unstructured free play should be encouraged to enhance enjoyment of sports, as well as to promote spontaneity and creativity.

Coaches, officials, parents, and program designers should view the preadolescent years as a time for teaching fundamental motor skills; developing fitness in a practical, safe, and gradual manner; and promoting desired attitudes and values. Practice sessions should incorporate these elements and allow time for unstructured play. The actual game or sporting event should also be managed in a manner that stresses these goals more than winning. To the extent possible, each child should receive equal playing time. Game rules should be modified to accommodate the child's need to learn or be adapted to age-appropriate skills or fitness. If possible, the child participants should be grouped according to size, skill, and maturational level rather than age. This is especially true at ages 11 to 14 years when some children are prepubertal and others are well into puberty.

The important objective for parents, coaches, and officials should be to enhance the child's self-image. Mastery of the sport (the athlete's performance within the activity) should be emphasized, instead of winning or pleasing others. Coaches and parents should assist children in setting realistic goals. Good effort should be praised, and mistakes should be met with encouragement and corrective instruction. Adults must clearly show that the child's worth is unrelated to the outcome of the game. Unconditional approval should be given for participating and having fun. Athletic programs should deemphasize playoffs and avoid all-star contests, excessive publicity, and elaborate recognition ceremonies that single out individuals. Ceremonies should recognize all participants.

Children may need assistance in maintaining a proper balance between sports and other life activities. Practice and game schedules should not

The recommendations in this statement do not indicate an exclusive course of treatment to be followed. Variations, taking into account individual circumstances, may be appropriate.

This statement has been approved by the Council on Child and Adolescent Health.

Reprint requests to Publications Department, American Academy of Pediatrics, 141 Northwest Point Blvd, PO Box 927, Elk Grove Village, IL 60009-0927.

interfere with school responsibilities, and family life should not revolve around the "child athlete" to the exclusion of other family members or needs.

The most effective means of instilling desirable attitudes and values is by role modeling. Coaches, officials, and parents must continuously monitor their own behavior to be sure it reflects the sharing, cooperation, honesty, and restraint they wish to see in the children. Coaches' lifestyle and behavior should reflect the health values they want to encourage in the children (weight control, fitness, good nutrition, and avoidance of alcohol, tobacco, and drugs).

Every program should provide adequate safeguards by requiring: (1) preparticipation physical examinations at least every 2 years; (2) warm-up procedures; (3) the availability of a medically trained person who is competent in recognizing significant injuries during practices and games of contact sports; (4) the establishment of policies for first-aid, referral of injured participants, treatment, rehabilitation, and certification for return to participation[2,3]; (5) suitable and well-maintained sports facilities; (6)appropriate protective equipment; (7) strict enforcement of rules concerning safety; and (8) a formal surveillance method to ensure that goals are met.

All coaches, whether paid or volunteer, should be required to review the guidelines and goals described above. In addition they should complete a coaching certification program that covers teaching techniques, basic sports skills, fitness, first-aid, sportsmanship, self-image enhancement, and motivation. Available certification programs for coaches include: (1) National Youth Sports Coaches Association, 2611 Old Okeechobee Rd, West Palm Beach, FL 33409 and (2) American Coaching Effectiveness Program, Human Kinetics Publishers, Inc, Box 5076, Champaign, IL 61820.

The pediatrician's role is to advise parents, schools, and community groups regarding these recommendations and to discuss these issues with parents as part of regular anticipatory guidance.

COMMITTEE ON SPORTS MEDICINE, 1988-1989
Michael A. Nelson, MD, Chairman
Barry Goldberg, MD
Suzanne B. Haefele, MD
Gregory L. Landry, MD
William L. Risser, MD

Liaison Representatives
Oded Bar-Or, MD, Canadian Paediatric Society
Richard Malacrea, National Athletic Trainers Association

AAP Section Liaison
David M. Orenstein, MD, Section on Diseases of the Chest
Arthur M. Pappas, MD, Section on Orthopaedics

COMMITTEE ON SCHOOL HEALTH, 1988-1989
Martin C. Ushkow, MD, Chairman
Beverley J. Bayes, MD
Philip R. Nader, MD
Jerry Newton, MD
Steven R. Poole, MD
Martin W. Sklaire, MD

Liaison Representatives
Jeffrey L. Black, MD, American School Health Association
Janice M. Fleszar, American Medical Association
Vivian Haines, National Association of School Nurses
Paul W. Jung, EdD, American Association of School Administrators
Patricia Lachelt, MS, National Association of Pediatric Nurse Associates and Practitioners
James H. Williams, National Education Association
Charles Zimont, MD, American Academy of Family Physicians

REFERENCES

1. American Academy of Pediatrics, Committees on Sports Medicine and School Health. Physical fitness and the schools. *Pediatrics.* 1987;80:449-450
2. American Academy of Pediatrics, Committee on Sports Medicine. *Sports Medicine: Health Care for Young Athletes.* Elk Grove Village, IL: American Academy of Pediatrics; 1983
3. American Academy of Pediatrics, Committee on School Health. *School Health: A Guide for Health Professionals.* Elk Grove Village, IL: American Academy of Pediatrics; 1987:182

Committee on Sports Medicine

Amenorrhea in Adolescent Athletes (RE9163)

A minority of female athletes participating in ballet, gymnastics, distance running, rowing, and cycling, as well as other sports activities, occasionally experience menstrual and associated physiologic changes. Women competing in the sports of ballet and gymnastics have been reported to have a particularly increased incidence of primary and secondary amenorrhea, decreased bone density, stress fractures, and symptoms of anorexia nervosa.[1-4] Results of several studies have indicated decreased levels of circulating estrogen as well as other metabolic changes.[1,3-7]

Research designed to determine the etiology of the amenorrhea and the associated changes has shown mixed results.

Low body fat cannot be linked in a causative fashion to hormonal changes or decreased levels of circulating estrogen. Early studies linking minimum body fat and menarche, as well as maintenance of regular menstrual cycles, have not been replicated.[8] However, measurement of percentage of body fat may be helpful in assessing the nutritional status of athletes.

Ballet and gymnastics are perceived by some to be activities that are stressful psychologically. Although stress has been shown to cause amenorrhea, studies to date have not demonstrated the presence of significantly increased levels compared with age-matched girls not participating in ballet and gymnastics.[9]

Some authors have postulated that tall, thin athletes who may be genetically at risk for delayed maturation are naturally attracted to these sports.[10] Some of the delays may relate to preselection. However, no evidence currently exists proving a definite relationship between preselection and the physiologic changes in these athletes.

There is an increased emphasis by athletes,

coaches, judges, and spectators on a slender physique for female gymnasts and ballet dancers. Several investigators have shown dietary intakes of adolescent ballerinas that are inadequate in calories, nutritional components, vitamins, and minerals.[2,6] The most common findings demonstrated in amenorrheic athletes are high intensity of exercise combined with poor nutritional status. Fasting and purging may be encouraged and anorexia nervosa or bulimia hidden in all athletic populations. Coaches need to be educated regarding the seriousness of these behaviors.

Recommendations for dealing with sports-related amenorrhea in adult women have included thorough physical examinations (including pelvic examinations) and endocrine evaluations, as well as estrogen and calcium supplementation.[11] Some of those recommendations are probably appropriate for adolescent athletes. Endocrine evaluation including studies of follicle-stimulating hormone, luteinizing hormone, thyroxine, prolactin, and estradiol should be performed if the athlete has menarche delayed greater than 1 year beyond the age of onset of menses of other female family members or if menses cease for 6 or more months after regular menses have been established. Pregnancy should always be ruled out early in the course of amenorrhea. In situations in which family history is not available, primary amenorrhea should be considered if menarche has not occurred by age 16 years and prompt evaluation initiated. Most adolescent athletes make adequate amounts of estrogen and will have withdrawal bleeding following progestin challenge. The use of supplemental estrogen in the young amenorrheic girl should not be routinely implemented. These young athletes should be encouraged to decrease the intensity of their exercise and to improve their nutritional intake. However, older athletes may be appropriately supplemented with estrogen.

The following recommendations are appropriate.

1. Preparticipation evaluations should include a focus on menstrual function and dietary practices.

2. Education and counseling should be provided to athletes, parents, and coaches regarding adequate intake of nutrients to maintain normal growth and development.[12]

PEDIATRICS (ISSN 0031 4005). Copyright © 1989 by the American Academy of Pediatrics.

3. During the active season, routine monitoring of menstrual function, growth velocity, dietary changes, weight changes, and, when possible, skin fold thickness should be performed.

4. The possibility of anorexia nervosa should be explored and when diagnosed treated in the same manner as anorexia nervosa in nonathletes.

5. Athletes whose diets provide less than 1200 mg/d of calcium should be supplemented to maintain an intake of 1200 to 1500 mg/d.

6. Amenorrheic athletes within 3 years of menarche should be counseled to decrease the intensity of exercise and improve their nutritional intake, especially protein. The use of hormonal therapy for these younger girls is generally not advised.

7. Because pregnancy continues to be a risk in amenorrheic athletes who are sexually active, the possibility of pregnancy should always be assessed as part of the evaluation.

8. The mature amenorrheic athlete (generally greater than 3 years past menarche or age 16 years), if found to be hypoestrogenemic, may benefit by receiving estrogen supplementation. Optimal therapy has yet to be determined, but supplementation with low-dose oral contraceptives (<50 μg of estrogen per day) is reasonable.

COMMITTEE ON SPORTS MEDICINE, 1986–1989
Michael A. Nelson, MD, Chairman, 1988–1989
Paul G. Dyment, MD, Chairman, 1986–1988
Barry Goldberg, MD
Suzanne B. Haefele, MD
Gregory L. Landry, MD
John J. Murray, MD
William L. Risser, MD

Liaison Representatives
Oded Bar-Or, MD, Canadian Paediatric Society

Richard Malacrea, National Athletic Trainers Association

AAP Section Liaison
David M. Orenstein, MD, Section on Diseases of the Chest
Arthur M. Pappas, MD, Section on Orthopaedics

REFERENCES

1. Athletic women, amenorrhea, and skeletal integrity, editorial. *Ann Intern Med.* 1985;102:258–260
2. Benson J, Gillien DM, Bourdet RD, et al. Inadequate nutrition and chronic calorie restriction in adolescent ballerinas. *Physician Sports Med.* 1985;13:79–90
3. Drinkwater BL, Nilson K, et al. Bone mineral content of amenorrheic and eumenorrheic athletes. *N Engl J Med.* 1984;311:277–281
4. Warren MP, Brooks-Gunn J, Hamilton LH, et al. Scoliosis and fractures in young ballet dancers: relation to delayed menarche and secondary amenorrhea. *N Engl J Med.* 1986;314:1348–1353
5. Loucks AB, Horvath SM. Athletic amenorrhea: a review. *Med Sci Sports Exer.* 1985;17:56–72
6. Braisted JR, Mellin L, Gong EJ, et al. The adolescent ballet dancer: nutritional practices and characteristics associated with anorexia nervosa. *J Adolesc Health Care.* 1985;6:365–371
7. Wilson C, Emans J, et al. The relationships of calculated percent body, sports participation, age and place of residence on menstrual patterns in healthy adolescent girls at an independent New England high school. *J Adolesc Health Care.* 1984;5:248–253
8. Frisch RE. Body fat, puberty and fertility. *Biol Rev.* 1984;59:161–188
9. Warren M. The effects of exercise on pubertal progression and reproduction function in girls. *J Clin Endocrinol Metab.* 1980;51:1150–1157
10. Malina RM. Menarche in athletes: a synthesis and hypothesis. *Ann Hum Biol.* 1983;10:1–24
11. Shangold MM. Causes, evaluation and management of athletic oligo-amenorrhea. *Med Clin North Am.* 1985;69:83–95
12. American Academy of Pediatrics, Committee on Nutrition. *Pediatric Nutrition Handbook.* 2nd ed. Elk Grove Village, IL: American Academy of Pediatrics; 1985

Committee on Sports Medicine

Infant Exercise Programs (RE8132)

Infant exercise programs are becoming abundant in the United States. In most programs, massage techniques, passive exercises, and holding an infant in various positions are used. Some programs involve the purchase of "exercise equipment." Promoters have claimed that participation by an infant in these programs will improve physical prowess.

In early infancy, the predominant neuromuscular responses are reflex in nature.[1] Most activity at this age can be attributed to an intrinsic arousal-seeking drive. Natural curiosity and the drive toward self-sufficiency motivate infants in virtually all activities.[2]

Providing a stimulating environment for an infant's development is extremely important. Environmental deprivation will impede the developmental progress of an infant. There is some evidence that conditioned responses can be elicited in the newborn period. However, there have been no data to suggest that structured programs or the promotion of conditioned responses will advance skills or provide any long-term benefit to normal infants.[3]

The bones of infants are more susceptible to trauma than those of older children and adults. The skeletal system of the child in the first year of life is less than optimally ossified.[4] Infants do not have the strength or reflexes necessary to protect themselves from external forces. The possibility exists that adults may inadvertently exceed the infant's physical limitations by using structured exercise programs.

Parents do not need specialized skills or equipment to provide an environment for the optimum development of their infant. An infant should be provided with opportunities for touching, holding, face-to-face contact, and minimally structured playing with safe toys. If these opportunities occur, an infant's intrinsic motivation will guide his or her individual developmental course.

Therefore, the AAP recommends that (1) structured infant exercise programs not be promoted as being therapeutically beneficial for the development of healthy infants and (2) parents be encouraged to provide a safe, nurturing, and minimally structured play environment for their infant.

COMMITTEE ON SPORTS MEDICINE, 1986–1988
Paul G. Dyment, MD, Chairman
Barry Goldberg, MD
Suzanne B. Haefele, MD
William L. Risser, MD
Michael A. Nelson, MD
John J. Murray, MD

Liaison Representatives
Oded Bar-Or, MD, Canadian Paediatric Society
Richard Malacrea, National Athletic
   Trainers Association

AAP Section Liaison
David M. Orenstein, MD, Section on
   Diseases of the Chest
Arthur M. Pappas, MD, Section on Orthopedics

This statement has been approved by the Council on Child and Adolescent Health.
The recommendations in this statement do not indicate an exclusive course of treatment or procedure to be followed. Variations, taking into account individual circumstances, may be appropriate.
PEDIATRICS (ISSN 0031 4005). Copyright © 1988 by the American Academy of Pediatrics.

REFERENCES

1. Rarick GL: Concepts of motor learning: Implications for skill development in children, in *Child in Sport and Physical Activity*: Selected papers presented at the National Conference Workshop, "The Child in Sport and Physical Activity." Baltimore, University Park Press, 1976, pp 203–217
2. Shephard RJ: Growth of motor skills: Motivating the child toward physical activity, in Shephard R (ed): *Physical Activity and Growth*. Chicago, Year Book Medical Publishers, 1982, pp 107–123, 233–245
3. Baldwin KM: Muscle development: Neonatal to adult. *Exercise Sport Sci Rev* 1984;12:1–19
4. Royer P: Growth and development of bony tissue, in Davis JA, Dobbiny J (ed): *Scientific Foundations of Paediatrics*. Philadelphia, WB Saunders Co, 1974, pp 376–398

Committee on Sports Medicine
Committee on Children With Disabilities

Exercise for Children Who Are Mentally Retarded (RE7096)

Recreation and exercise are important for all children, regardless of their mental capacity. A physician's recommendation about athletic activity for a mentally retarded child, as with any child, must take into account the child's size, coordination, degree of physical fitness, physical maturity, physical health, and motivation. It is also important to consider physical problems that may be specific to a child or to a child's condition (eg, atlantoaxial instability in a child with Down syndrome). In some communities, there is a tendency to exclude mentally retarded children from exercise programs. Because children who are mentally retarded frequently have poor coordination, it may be more difficult for them to be physically active in the "usual" programs. This can contribute to lassitude and excessive weight gain.

ROLE OF PEDIATRICIAN

Parents of mentally retarded children are often confused and uncertain about what to expect from their children. Some tend to restrict their youngster from physical activities; others may push their child at too rapid a pace. Most parents are eager for guidance to help determine what is best for their child. Pediatricians are in a unique position to advise these parents. They have knowledge of the family and are aware of the emotional and personal needs and the physical capabilities of the child.

BENEFITS OF PARTICIPATION IN SPORTS

Mentally retarded children may have greater success in individual and dual sports than in team sports. Competition is often highly motivating, and it may be a means of promoting self-satisfaction as well as developing muscles and coordination. The Special Olympics has shown that retarded children can successfully compete against each other. Regardless of their intellectual capacity, children have a wide range of athletic ability. Some mentally retarded children are well coordinated; some highly intelligent children are clumsy.

There are mutual benefits when retarded children participate in noncompetitive sports with children of normal intelligence. One important benefit is the educational opportunities for the "normal" children to learn about disabilities and their effects on their mentally retarded peers. It should be remembered when planning activities that there is some correlation between developmental level and persistence, attention span, emotional control, and understanding the rules of the game. Children who are mentally retarded usually perform best and enjoy themselves most with children of the same developmental level, not necessarily children of the same chronologic age.

Children elicit more interest in games than in simple exercises. Game rules may be changed so that most of the children are interacting most of the time; this is often necessary because retarded children may have a short attention span. In addition, participation with other children may enhance youngsters' self-esteem and help them learn cooperation. Keeping records of personal improvement, counting, and similar intellectual activity on the part of mentally retarded children may provide ancillary intellectual benefits from participation in vigorous physical efforts.[1]

Practical suggestions about facilities, equipment, playground markings, fitness activities, and selected exercise are available.[1] Information about physical activity programs for the mentally retarded is also available from the American Alliance for Health, Physical Education, Recreation, and Dance,[2] formerly known as the American Association for Health, Physical Education, and Recreation.[3,4] In addition, the Kennedy Foundation also

This statement has been approved by the Council on Child and Adolescent Health. The recommendations in this statement do not indicate an exclusive course of treatment or procedure to be followed. Variations, taking into account individual circumstances, may be appropriate.
PEDIATRICS (ISSN 0031 4005). Copyright © 1987 by the American Academy of Pediatrics.

provides information about specific model programs, such as the Special Olympics Program (Special Olympics, Inc, Joseph P. Kennedy, Jr, Foundation, 719 13th St, NW, Washington, DC 20005). Many programs for the mentally retarded are best planned at the community level. Communities that take on this responsibility have the added opportunity to provide activities that enable retarded and nonretarded children to participate together and thus decrease some of the problems created by isolation of the mentally retarded. The general population, especially children, lacks knowledge about mental retardation and usually does not have the opportunity to develop the appropriate understanding of its mentally retarded peers. Children who are mentally retarded are sometimes rejected because they lack personal and social skills, partly as a result of their relative isolation from other children. Interacting with children of normal intelligence through sports activities helps mentally retarded children to develop these personal and social skills as well as improving their physical well-being.

SUMMARY

Pediatricians should encourage participation in exercise and athletic programs for mentally retarded children. The right program can be a therapeutic tool resulting in better weight management, development of physical coordination, maintenance of cardiopulmonary fitness, and improved self-esteem.

COMMITTEE ON SPORTS MEDICINE,
1986–1987
Paul G. Dyment, MD, Chairman
Barry Goldberg, MD
Suzanne B. Haefele, MD
John J. Murray, MD
Michael A. Nelson, MD

Liaison Representatives
Oded Bar-Or, MD, Canadian
Paediatric Society

Richard Malacrea, MD, National
Athletic Trainers Association
AAP Section Liaison
David M. Orenstein, MD,
Section on Diseases of the Chest
Arthur M. Pappas, MD,
Section on Orthopaedics

COMMITTEE ON CHILDREN WITH DISABILITIES,
1986–1987
Herbert J. Cohen, MD, Chairman
Robert F. Biehl, MD
Lucy S. Crain, MD
Julian S. Haber, MD
Alfred Healy, MD
Avrum L. Katcher, MD
Sonya G. Oppenheimer, MD
James M. Perrin, MD

Liaison Representatives
Thomas R. Bellamy, PhD, Director
Office of Special Education Programs
Ross Hays, MD, American Academy
of Physical Medicine and Rehabilitation
Andrea Knight, Association for Retarded
Citizens

Section Liaison
Barry Russman, MD, Section
on Neurology
Bram Bernstein, MD, Section
on Rheumatology

REFERENCES

1. Cratty BJ: Improving the physical fitness of retardates, in Pearson PH, Williams CE (eds): *Physical Therapy Services in the Developmental Disabilities.* Springfield, IL, Charles C Thomas Publisher, 1972, p 338
2. *Aerobic Fitness for the Moderately Retarded.* Reston, VA, American Alliance for Health, Physical Education, Recreation, and Dance, 1980, vol 5
3. *Annotated Research Bibliography in Physical Education, Recreation and Psychomotor Function of Mentally Retarded Person.* Washington, DC, American Association for Health, Physical Education and Recreation, 1975
4. *Physical Activities for the Mentally Retarded: Ideas for Instruction.* Washington, DC, American Association for Health, Physical Education and Recreation, 1968

Committee on Sports Medicine
Committee on School Health

Physical Fitness and the Schools   (RE7097)

During the last decade our concept of what "physical fitness" means has undergone a major change. Traditionally the "physically fit" child was one who had obvious motor (or athletic) abilities, ordinarily defined by such parameters as muscle strength, agility, speed, and power. But the high levels of power, speed, and agility necessary for success in most competitive sports have little or no relevance in the daily lives of most adults. Today, the words "physical fitness" imply optimal functioning of all physiologic systems of the body, particularly the cardiovascular, pulmonary, and musculoskeletal systems.[1]

DEFINING PHYSICAL FITNESS

Physical fitness is now considered to include five components: muscle strength and endurance, flexibility, body composition (ie, degree of fatness), and cardiorespiratory endurance. Good cardiorespiratory endurance may be associated with a lessened chance of disability or death due to cardiovascular disease. Schools in the United States have traditionally emphasized sports such as football and baseball, both of which require agility and skill but are not particularly fitness enhancing. Aerobic activities (eg, activities requiring maintenance of 75% of maximal heart rate for 20 to 25 minutes), if performed at least three times a week, can lead to enhanced cardiorespiratory endurance. This improvement in fitness can be achieved by swimming, running, bicycling, field hockey, aerobic dancing, fast walking, etc.

SCHOOL PROGRAMS

Unfortunately, just as the understanding of the importance of health-related physical fitness has

become widespread, our ability to direct youth activities toward fitness is being countered by several new pressures: (1) Financial strains may lead public school systems to reduce physical education budgets. (2) Widespread disenchantment with the results of several decades of "progressive education experiments" has resulted in pressures on school administrators to do away with "frills" and to return to the "basics"; this might lead to deemphasis of physical education classes. (3) Children and adolescents are lured to watch television in their spare time. (4) Finally, most aerobic activities (eg, running, swimming laps) are not perceived to be pleasurable, and it is extremely difficult to motivate children to begin a lifelong habit of maintaining a high degree of physical fitness if this involves repeated endurance physical activities.

American children do not perform well on standardized tests of fitness.[2,3] In one 1985 study, 40% of boys 6 to 12 years of age could not do more than one pull-up, nor could 70% of girls of all ages.[2] In this 1985 study, general levels of physical fitness were compared with levels found in a 1975 study of randomly selected students; in general, there had been no improvement in physical fitness levels. The National Children and Youth Fitness Study of the US Department of Health and Human Services compared body composition values for children in 1985 with values for a group of children tested in the 1960s; it was concluded that on the average children are fatter now.[3]

ROLE OF PEDIATRICIAN

Because financial support for fitness programs in the schools is unlikely to increase in the foreseeable future, and television is unlikely to become less attractive, we must anticipate the probability that our children's degree of physical fitness will decline. Pediatricians must acquaint themselves with this problem and appeal to their local school boards to maintain, if not increase, the school's physical education program of physical fitness. School programs should emphasize the so-called lifetime athletic activities such as cycling, swimming, and ten-

This statement has been approved by the Council on Child and Adolescent Health. The recommendations in this statement do not indicate an exclusive course of treatment or procedure to be followed. Variations, taking into account individual circumstances, may be appropriate.
PEDIATRICS (ISSN 0031 4005). Copyright © 1987 by the American Academy of Pediatrics.

nis. Schools should decrease time spent teaching the skills used in team sports such as football, basketball, and baseball. Physical fitness activities at school should promote a lifelong habit of aerobic exercise. During anticipatory guidance sessions, pediatricians should encourage parents to see that all family members are involved in fitness-enhancing physical activities, so that these activities become an integral part of the family's life-style.

COMMITTEE ON SPORTS MEDICINE, 1986–1987
Paul G. Dyment, MD, Chairman
Barry Goldberg, MD
Suzanne B. Haefele, MD
John J. Murray, MD
Michael A. Nelson, MD

Liaison Representatives
Oded Bar-Or, MD, Canadian
    Paediatric Society
Richard Malacrea, MD, National
    Athletic Trainers Association

AAP Section Liaison
David M. Orenstein, MD, Section
    on Diseases of the Chest
Arthur M. Pappas, MD, Section
    on Orthopaedics

COMMITTEE ON SCHOOL HEALTH, 1986–1987
Joseph R. Zanga, MD, Chairman
Michael A. Donlan, MD
Jerry Newton, MD
Maxine M. Sehring, MD
Martin W. Sklaire, MD
Martin C. Ushkow, MD

Liaison Representatives
Jeffrey L. Black, MD, American
    School Health Association
Patricia Lachelt, National Association
    of Pediatric Nurse Associates and
    Practitioners
Nick Staresinic, PhD, American Association
    of School Administrators
Bonnie Wilford, PhD, American
    Medical Association
Charles Zimont, MD, American
    Academy of Family Physicians

REFERENCES

1. Pate RR: A new definition of youth fitness. *Phys Sports Med* 1983;11:77–83
2. Reiff GG, Dixon WR, Jacoby D, et al: *Youth Physical Fitness in 1985.* Washington, DC, President's Council on Physical Fitness and Sports, 1985
3. US Department of Health and Human Services: The National Children and Youth Fitness Study. *J Phys Educ Recreation Dance* January 1985, pp 44–90

American Academy of Pediatrics

Policy Statement:
Infant swimming programs (RE5045)

There is little justification for infant "swimming" or water adjustment programs. However, a growing number of programs promoting infant swimming can be found across the country, and they claim a variety of benefits such as enhancing parent-child communication and other "values". Giardiasis transmission[2] and water intoxication with seizures[3-8] make these programs somewhat hazardous. It is unlikely that infants can be made "water safe"; in fact, the parents of these infants may develop a false sense of security if they believe that their infant can "swim" a few strokes.

Recommendations

The American Academy of Pediatrics, in recognizing the increasing popularity of swimming programs for infants and the enjoyment of the parent and infant who share this activity, makes the following recommendations:

1. A parent who enrolls an infant in a water adjustment program, should understand and accept the risks.

2. To reduce these risks, the program should follow the national YMCA guidelines which include[9]; prohibiting total submersion, maintaining an appropriate water temperature, and providing measures to control fecal contamination.

3. The swimming experience of each infant should be on a one-to-one basis with a parent or responsible adult. Organized group swimming instruction should be reserved for children more than three years of age.

4. Instruction should be carried out by qualified instructors familiar with infant CPR techniques in properly maintained pools.

5. Infants with known medical problems should recieve their physician's approval before participation.

6. Studies of the frequency of risks to infants from water adjustment programs should be carried out as soon as possible.

This statement has been approved by the Council on Child and Adolescent Health. ∎

Committee on Sports Medicine (1984-85)
Paul G. Dyment, M.D., Chairman
Eugene F. Luckstead, M.D.
John J. Murray, M.D.
Michael A. Nelson, M.D.
Nathan J. Smith, M.D.

Liaison Representatives;
James H. Moller, M.D.
Section on Cardiology
Frederick W. Baker, M.D.
Canadian Paediatric Society
Richard Malacrea
National Athletic Trainers Association
David M. Orenstein, M.D.
Section on Diseases of the Chest
Arthur M. Pappas, M.D.
Section on Orthopaedics

References
1. Committee on Pediatric Aspects of Physical Fitness, Recreation, and Sports: Swimming Instructions for Infants. Pediatrics 1980; 65:847.
2. Harter L, Frost F, Grunerfelder G: Giardiasis in an infant and toddler swim class. AM. J. Pub. Hlth. 1984; 74:155.
3. Bennett HJ, Wegner T, Fields A: Acute hyponatremia and seizures in an infant after a swimming lesson. Pediatrics 1983; 72:125-127.
4. Geda MW: Texas Medicine (letter) 1982; 78:6.
5. Goldberg GN, Lightner ES, Morgan W, et al: Infantile water intoxication after a swimming lesson. Pediatrics 1982; 70:599.
6. Kropp RM, Schwartz JF: Water intoxication from swimming. Journal of Pediatrics 1982; 101:947.
7. Pediatric Notes 1981; 4:59-60.
8. Pediatric Notes 1981; 4:88.
9. YMCA Guidelines for Infant Swiming, Division of Aquatics, YMCA of the USA, 101 N. Wacker Drive, Chicago, IL 60606, 1984.

Committee on Sports Medicine

UNDER REVISION

Atlantoaxial Instability in Down Syndrome (RE4910)

Some issues related to participation in certain sports by persons with Down syndrome require clarification.

Since 1965 there have been occasional reports about a condition described at various times as instability, subluxation, or dislocation of the articulation of the first and second cervical vertebrae (atlantoaxial joint) among persons with Down syndrome.[1-15] This condition has also been found in patients with rheumatoid arthritis,[16,17] abnormalities of the odontoid process of the second cervical vertebra,[4,5,12,13,15] and various forms of dwarfism.[18] Atlantoaxial (C-1, C-2) instability has not attracted general attention because clinical manifestations are rare and the condition is limited to a small portion of the population. The incidence of atlantoaxial instability among persons with Down syndrome has been reported by various observers to be 10% to 20%.[2,9,15] When atlantoaxial instability results in subluxation or dislocation of C-1 and C-2, the spinal cord also may be injured. This is a rare but serious complication.

In March 1983, the Special Olympics, Inc, sponsors of a nationwide competitive athletic program for developmentally disabled persons, without prior announcement, mandated for participants with Down syndrome special precautions to prevent serious neurologic consequences from stress on the head and neck in sports competition.[19] Although thousands of persons with Down syndrome have taken part in sports events during the 15-year history of the Special Olympics without a known occurrence of neurologic complications due to participation, the new directive requires all persons with Down syndrome who wish to participate in certain sports that might involve stress on the head and neck (gymnastics, diving, pentathlon, butterfly stroke in swimming, diving start in swimming, high jump, soccer, and warm-up exercises that place undue stress on the head and neck muscles) to have

---

This statement has been approved by the Council on Child and Adolescent Health.

PEDIATRICS (ISSN 0031 4005). Copyright © 1984 by the American Academy of Pediatrics.

a medical examination, lateral-view roentgenograms of the upper cervical region in full flexion and extension, and certification by a physician that the examination did not reveal atlantoaxial instability or neurologic disorder. Failure either to comply or to have medical certification would result in exclusion from the above-specified sports.

Parents, physicians, and sports authorities were understandably surprised by the immediacy of the edict. Many parents were resentful because of the short time for screening, the cost of the examinations, and discovery that most physicians did not know about the directive or were not aware of the atlantoaxial syndrome. Some radiologists were not familiar with exact procedures for screening. In general, physicians were perplexed by the sudden concern about a condition that had never been a problem among the largest group of disabled participants during 15 seasons of the Special Olympics.

There are no national statistics to confirm the extent of screening in 1983, but valiant efforts were made to comply with the directive during the 6-week interval allowed for the procedures. It has been stated that there were no reported casualties due to atlantoaxial instability in the Special Olympics last year. However, some participants were barred from the specified events.

Atlantoaxial (C-1, C-2) instability is a manifestation of the generalized poor muscle tone and joint laxity commonly found in persons with Down syndrome. The instability is due to (1) laxity of the transverse ligament that holds the odontoid process of the axis (C-2) in place against the inner aspect of the anterior arch of the atlas (C-1), maintaining integrity of the C-1, C-2 articulation or (2) abnormalities of the odontoid, such as hypoplasia, malformation, or complete absence.[4,5,9,13,15] These conditions allow some leeway between the odontoid and the atlas, especially during flexion and extension of the neck. This results in a "loose joint." In extreme cases, the first cervical vertebra slips forward and the spinal cord is vulnerable to compression by the odontoid process of C-2 anteriorly or by the arch of C-1 posteriorly.

Measurement of the distance between the odontoid process and the anterior arch of the atlas on lateral roentgenograms in the neutral, flexion, and extension positions is the only way to detect atlantoaxial instability.[9,14,20]

Although simple laxity and instability seldom lead to subluxation or dislocation, it has become apparent, as physicians learn more about atlantoaxial instability, that the latent condition must be viewed as a factor predisposing to neurologic complications. Detection of an abnormal space between the odontoid and the anterior arch of the atlas is a signal for precautionary measures to avoid hyperflexion or hyperextension of the neck and extreme rotation of the head.

The neurologic manifestations of spinal compression from the above causes include fatigue in walking, gait disturbance, progressive clumsiness and incoordination, spasticity, hyperreflexia, clonus, toe-extensor reflex, and other upper motor neuron and posterior column signs and symptoms from compression of the spinal cord. Onset of neck pain, head tilt, and torticollis in Down syndrome are indicative of malposition of the odontoid. Development, and particularly, progression of these neurologic signs or symptoms in a person with Down syndrome suggest atlantoaxial subluxation. Strenuous activity should be curtailed and diagnosis and management undertaken promptly.

It is very likely that many schools, recreation and rehabilitation programs, and camps in which developmentally disabled persons are enrolled will follow the example of the Special Olympics in requiring careful screening of all persons with Down syndrome before participation in activities that could result in flexion and hyperextension is permitted. Undoubtedly, pediatricians, other primary care physicians, and radiologists will be called upon to screen and authorize participation.

RECOMMENDATIONS

The Committee on Sports Medicine, after consultation with the Sections on Neurology, Orthopaedics, and Radiology, recommends the following guidelines:

1. All children with Down syndrome who wish to participate in sports that involve possible trauma to the head and neck should have lateral-view roentgenograms of the cervical region in neutral, flexion, and extension positions within the patient's tolerance before beginning training or competition. This recommendation applies to all participants in the high-risk sports who have not previously had normal findings on cervical roentgenograms.

Some physicians may prefer to screen all patients with Down syndrome routinely at 5 to 6 years of age to rule out atlantoaxial instability.

2. When the distance between the odontoid process of the axis and the anterior arch of the atlas exceeds 4.5 mm or the odontoid is abnormal, there should be restrictions on sports that involve trauma to the head and neck, and the patient should be followed up at regular intervals.

3. At the present time, repeated roentgenograms are not indicated for those who have previously had normal findings. Indications for repeated roentgenograms will be defined by research.

4. Persons with atlantoaxial subluxation or dislocation and neurologic signs or symptoms should be restricted in all strenuous activities, and operative stabilization of the cervical spine should be considered.[21-23]

5. Persons with Down syndrome who have no evidence of atlantoaxial instability may participate in all sports. Follow-up is not required unless musculoskeletal or neurologic signs or symptoms develop.

COMMITTEE ON SPORTS MEDICINE, 1983–1984
Thomas E. Shaffer, MD, Chairman
Paul G. Dyment, MD
Eugene F. Luckstead, MD
John J. Murray, MD
Nathan J. Smith, MD

Liaison Representatives
James H. Moller, MD
   Section on Cardiology
David M. Orenstein, MD
   Section on Diseases of the Chest
Arthur M. Pappas, MD
   Section on Orthopaedics
Frederick W. Baker, MD
   Canadian Paediatric Society
Richard Malacrea
   National Athletic Trainers Association

Consultants
E. Dennis Lyne, MD, Chairman
   Section on Orthopaedics
Gerald Erenberg, MD, Chairman
   Section on Neurology
Bruce R. Parker, MD, Chairman
   Section on Radiology
Albert C. Fremont, Chairman
   Committee on Children with Disabilities

REFERENCES

1. Tishler JM, Martel W: Dislocation of the atlas in mongolism: Preliminary report. Radiology 1965;84:904–906
2. Martel W, Tishler JM: Observations on the spine in mongolism. AJR 1966;97:630–638
3. Dzenitis AJ: Spontaneous atlanto-axial dislocation in a mongoloid with spinal cord compression: Case report. J Neurosurg 1966;25:458–460

4. Sherk HH, Nicholson JT: Rotatory atlanto-axial dislocation associated with ossiculum terminale and mongolism. *J Bone Joint Surg* 1969;51-A:957-963
5. Martel W, Uyham R, Stimson CW: Subluxation of the atlas causing spinal cord compression in a case of Down's syndrome with a "manifestation of an occipital vertebra." *Radiology* 1969;93:839-840
6. Gerard Y, Segal P, Bedoucha JS: L' instabilite de l'atlas sur l'axis dans le mongolisme. *Presse Med* 1971;79:573-575
7. Aung MH: Atlanto-axial dislocation in Down's syndrome: Report of a case with spinal cord compression and review of the literature. *Bull Los Angeles Neurol Soc* 1973;39:197-201
8. Finerman GAM, Sakai D, Weingarten S: Atlanto-axial dislocation with spinal cord compression in a mongoloid child: A case report. *J Bone Joint Surg* 1976;58-A:408-409
9. Semine AA, Ertel AN, Goldberg MJ, et al: Cervical spine instability in children with Down syndrome (trisomy 21). *J Bone Joint Surg* 1978;60-A:649-652
10. Whaley WJ, Gray WD: Atlantoaxial dislocation and Down's syndrome. *Can Med Assoc J* 1980;123:35-37
11. Shield LK, Dickens DRV, Jensen F: Atlanto-axial dislocation with spinal cord compression in Down syndrome. *Aust Paediatr J* 1981;17:114-116
12. Hungerford GD, Akkaraju V, Rawe SE, et al: Altanto-occipital and atlanto-axial dislocations with spinal cord compression in Down's syndrome: A case report and review of the literature. *Br J Radiol* 1981;54:758-761
13. Hreidarsson S, Magram G, Singer H: Symptomatic atlantoaxial dislocation in Down syndrome. *Pediatrics* 1982;69:568-571
14. Coria F, Quintana F, Villalba M, et al: Craniocervical ab-
normalities in Down's syndrome. *Dev Med Child Neurol* 1983;25:252-255
15. Pueschel SM, Scola FH, Perry CD: Atlanto-axial instability in children with Down syndrome. *Pediatr Radiol* 1981;10:129-132
16. Stevens JC, Cartlidge NEF, Saunders M, et al: Atlanto-axial subluxation and cervical myelopathy in rheumatoid arthritis. *Q J Med* 1971;40:391-408
17. Herring JA: Cervical instability in Down's syndrome and juvenile rheumatoid arthritis. *J Pediatr Orthop* 1982;2:205-207
18. Kopits SE, Perovic MN, McKusick V, et al: Congenital atlanto-axial dislocations in various forms of dwarfism. *J Bone Joint Surg* 1972;54:1349-1350
19. *Special Olympics Bulletin: Participation by individuals with Down syndrome who suffer from atlantoaxial dislocation condition.* Washington, DC, Special Olympics Inc, March 31, 1983
20. Locke GR, Gardner JI, Van Epps EF: Atlas-dens interval (ADI) in children: A survey based on 200 normal cervical spines. *AJR* 1966;135-140
21. Giblin PE, Micheli LJ: Management of atlanto-axial subluxation with neurologic involvement in Down syndrome: A report of two cases and review of the literature. *Clin Orthop* 1979;140:66-71
22. Spierings ELH, Braakman R: The management of os odontoideum: Analysis of 37 cases. *J Bone Joint Surg* 1982;64-B:422-428
23. Diamond LS, Lynne D, Sigman B: Orthopedic disorders in patients with Down's syndrome. *Orthop Clin North Am* 1981;12:57-71

AMERICAN ACADEMY OF PEDIATRICS

**Committee on Children with Handicaps and
Committee on Sports Medicine**

Sports and the Child with Epilepsy (RE2218)

The 1968 statement of the Committee on Children with Handicaps, "The Epileptic Child and Competitive School Athletics," is restated with considerable modification.

The responsibility for weighing the risks involved in athletic participation should be shared by the parents, the physician, and the child. Such risks should be weighed against the psychological trauma resulting from unnecessary restriction of physical activities. Parents should participate in all decisions. To the degree appropriate to the age and judgment of the child, his or her wishes should be considered. The young athlete must be taught that there is a risk of injury and he or she should be prepared to impose voluntary restrictions on physical activity depending upon the nature and frequency of seizures.

Proper medical management, good seizure control, and proper supervision are essential if children with epilepsy are to participate fully in physical education programs and interscholastic athletics. Common sense dictates that situations in which a seizure could cause a *dangerous* fall should be avoided. These situations include rope climbing, activity on parallel bars, and high diving. Swimming should be supervised; no competitive underwater swimming is acceptable. Participation in contact or collision sports should be given individual consideration according to the specific problem of the athlete. Epilepsy per se should not exclude a child from hockey, baseball, football, basketball, and wrestling.

Physicians who take care of childen who are involved in athletics should realize that in today's culture, sports and athletic activity are extremely important to young people and that unnecessarily strict interpretation of medical conditions may in fact do more harm than good.

COMMITTEE ON CHILDREN WITH HANDICAPS, 1982-1983
Albert C. Fremont, MD, Chairman
Herbert J. Cohen, MD
James W. Coker, Jr, MD
Alfred Healy, MD
David W. MacFarlane, MD
Bernard Weisskopf, MD

J. Albert Browder, MD, ARC-USA
Jane C. S. Perrin, MD, AAPM
Barry Russman, MD
   Section on Neurology
Herman Saettler, EdD

COMMITTEE ON SPORTS MEDICINE, 1982-1983
Thomas E. Shaffer, MD, Chairman
Paul G. Dyment, MD
Eugene F. Luckstead, MD
John J. Murray, MD
Nathan J. Smith, MD

Frederick W. Baker, MD
   Canadian Paediatric Society
Henry Levison, MD
   Section on Diseases of the Chest
James H. Moller, MD
   Section on Cardiology
Arthur M. Pappas, MD
   Section on Orthopaedics
Richard Malacrea, NATA

This statement has been approved by the Council on Child and Adolescent Health.
PEDIATRICS (ISSN 0031 4005). Copyright © 1983 by the American Academy of Pediatrics.

REFERENCES

Bennett PB, Elliott DH: *The Physiology and Medicine of Diving and Compressed Air Work*, ed 2. Baltimore, Williams & Wilkins, 1975

Committee on Children with Handicaps, American Academy of Pediatrics: The epileptic child and competitive school athletics. *Pediatrics* 1968;42:700

Committee on the Medical Aspects of Sports, American Medical Association: Epileptics and contact sports. *JAMA* 1974;229:820

Committee on School Health, American Academy of Pediatrics: *School Health: A Guide for Health Professionals*. American Academy of Pediatrics, Evanston, IL, 1981

Korezyn AD: Participation of epileptic patients in sports. *J Sports Med* 1979;19:195

Livingston S, Berman W: Participation of the epileptic child in contact sports. *J Sports Med* 1974;2:170

Pearn J, Bart R, Yamaoka R: Drowning risks to epileptic children: A study from Hawaii. *Br Med J* 1978;2:1284

AMERICAN ACADEMY OF PEDIATRICS

Committee on Drugs and Committee on Sports Medicine

Dimethyl Sulfoxide (DMSO)   (RE0337)

Dimethyl sulfoxide (DMSO) is an industrial solvent that has become a legend in its own time. In 1963, Dr Stanley Jacob introduced DMSO to reduce the swelling and pain of arthritis. Quickly, a wide variety of unsubstantiated claims were made, and enthusiasm apparently precluded careful studies.

In fact, the compound has a number of interesting pharmacologic properties that may be beneficial to patients. Its ability to penetrate intact skin, carrying a variety of chemicals, offers hope for eliminating many painful injections; its inhibition of certain prostaglandins offers hope that various inflammatory diseases may be suppressed; its local analgesic properties may reduce cutaneous pain from burns and injuries; its ability to dissolve compounds such as amyloid and collagen might be harnessed; and DMSO's ability to reduce increased intracranial pressure in head injuries could reduce morbidity if not mortality.

But research has not yet demonstrated that the potential of DMSO can be safely fulfilled. Clinical research was suspended in 1965 when injury to the lens was found in animals, but inasmuch as no human injury was detected, limited studies were permitted again in 1968. Asked for an opinion in 1972, the National Academy of Sciences stated that the compound should remain an investigational drug. During this period many papers detailed anecdotal results of cutaneous, intravenous, or oral use, and in 1978 the FDA approved Rimso (50% solution of DMSO) for the treatment of interstitial cystitis, the only approved use of the drug today. In the same year the Arthritis Advisory Committee to the Food and Drug Administration rejected the new drug application approval of DMSO based on the submitted studies. The committee requested that the National Institute of Health Center for Cooperative Studies of Rheumatic Diseases perform a controlled study of DMSO treatment of cutaneous ulcers in scleroderma, a study now underway. Other work, in progress or completed, includes studies on head injury, strain and sprain, and transcutaneous carrier properties.

Research to date has shown that the use of DMSO has a number of unpleasant features. Among these is "musty, garlicky" breath odor in about 80% of patients within minutes of skin application; this odor also permeates clothing and furniture in contact with skin to which DMSO has been applied. Local skin sensitivity with erythema and ulceration is common. In addition, the treatment regimen (immersing a part of the body in a DMSO solution several times a day for five to ten minutes) is difficult to maintain.

A further difficulty with DMSO is the nature of the products currently available, "veterinary" and "industrial" strengths. Veterinary DMSO, usually a 90% solution, because of its heavy concentration causes greater cutaneous toxicity. The industrial solution is usually even stronger, and the manufacturer makes no claim regarding absence of contaminants. Although no cases of poisoning through contamination have been substantiated, the lining of storage containers could contaminate the DMSO. If the skin is contaminated with dirt or chemicals, it is important to remember that DMSO probably will carry these compounds through the skin and into the circulation.

Pediatricians are likely to be asked by parents and athletic coaches whether DMSO is safe and effective for the treatment of sprains and strains. The answer is that the DMSO products currently available (veterinary and industrial) cannot be considered safe for human use and that effectiveness for this purpose has not been established.

This statement has been approved by the Council on Child and Adolescent Health.
PEDIATRICS (ISSN 0031 4005). Copyright © 1983 by the American Academy of Pediatrics.

American Academy Of Pediatrics Policy Statement

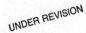

Horseback Riding And Related Injuries (RE2407)

Horseback riding accidents are a serious cause of head injuries with resultant death or permanent residual defects, and they are one of the leading causes of injuries from recreational activities.[1-3] This paper will recommend steps for preventing and/or lessening the severity of horseback riding-related injuries.

The Committee commends the American Horse Shows Association and the American Horse Council for their concern for horseback riding safety practices and for their participation in the horseback riding-related accident studies which are currently being conducted. Final recommendations will be made by the Committee for safer equestrian activities from the data being collected. However, the risks have been sufficiently defined and the scope of the problem of horseback riding-related injuries is large enough that preliminary recommendations can be made.

1. Educational programs should be given to parents, riding instructors, show organizers, and managers emphasizing the risks in horseback riding and methods to minimize them. Although 90 per cent of all horseback riding-related injuries occur in amateurs,[4] enough risks are inherent in this activity for persons of all ability levels that earnest attempts can be made to lessen them. Parents should be urged to see that the horses their children ride are within their capabilities.

2. A satisfactory, protective hat must be developed for each type of riding activity and worn when riding or preparing to ride. The Snell Foundation Equestrian Standards[5] for protective headgear have been developed by using laboratory testing models for protection against impact and penetration as well as strap strength for holding the helmet in place. Until further testing is completed, the manufacturers of protective headgear should meet the standards developed by acceptable testing organizations[6] — with medical input — and the headgear should be made so it can be worn with the appropriate riding dress: hunt, saddle seat, western, or costume.

3. All riding schools, horse shows, rodeos, and other events in which young persons participate with horses should require that a protective hat be worn during the activity. Points should be counted against the rider or the rider should be disqualified for awards if this requirement is not met.

References

[1] Mahaley, M.S., Jr., and Seaber, A.V.: "Accident and Safety Considerations of Horseback Riding," *Proceedings of the 18th Conference of Medical Aspects of Sports, Dallas, June 26, 1976,* pp. 37-45. Chicago: American Medical Association, 1977.

[2] Gleave, J.R.W.: "The Impact of Sports on a Neurosurgical Unit," Institute of Sports Medicine, Department of Neurological Surgery and Neurology, Cambridge Health District, Addenbrokes Hospital, Cambridge, England.

[3] Phillips, G.H., and Stuckey, W.E.: "Accidents to Rural Ohio People Occurring During Recreational Activities," *Extension Bulletin MM-295, Research Circular 166.* Wooster, Ohio: Ohio Agricultural Research and Development Center, January, 1969.

[4] Grossman, J.A., Kulund, D.N., Miller, C.W., Winn, H.R., and Hodge, R.H., Jr.: "Equestrian Injuries: Results of a Prospective Study," *JAMA 240:17, 1978.*

[5] Snell Memorial Foundation, George G. Snively, M.D., Director of Research, Sacramento, California.

[6] Such as NOCSAE, ASTM, and the Snell Foundation.

This statement has been reviewed and approved by the AAP Council on Child and Adolescent Health.

Committee on Pediatric Aspects of Physical Fitness, Recreation, and Sports
Thomas G. Flynn, M.D., Chairman
John H. Kennell, M.D.
Robert N. McLeod, Jr., M.D.
Thomas E. Shaffer, M.D.
William B. Strong, M.D.
Melvin L. Thornton, M.D.
Clemens, W. Van Rooy, M.D.

Liaison Members
Lucille Burkett, AAHPERD
Richard Malacrea, National Athletic Trainers Assn.
Kaye E. Wilkins, M.D., Section on Orthopaedics

Date of approval by AAP Executive Committee: October 1980.
Date of publication: December 1980.

AMERICAN ACADEMY OF PEDIATRICS

Committee on Pediatric Aspects of Physical Fitness, Recreation, and Sports

UNDER REVISION

Fitness in the Preschool Child (RE2208)

Achieving fitness is a way of life, not a fad or a brief change in one's way of doing things. And, an early start is imperative. A flaw in our present system of health care is the emphasis on evaluation of anatomic or organic soundness and the presence or absence of disease—with less regard for the quality of physiologic function. In other words, dynamic performance is frequently ignored after the organic condition has been determined. An infant or child may well be regarded as healthy with the proper immunizations and absence of disease. But, is he/she able to meet daily tasks, recreational activities, and unforeseen emergencies with vigor and enthusiasm and without undue fatigue? Is he/she making adequate use of the musculoskeletal and cardiopulmonary systems?

Lack of encouragement to exercise in early life is reflected in the National Adult Physical Fitness Survey conducted by the President's Council on Physical Fitness in 1972. This study showed that 45% of all adult Americans do not engage in physical activity for the purpose of exercise. However, 63% of these nonexercisers said they believed they had enough exercise; only 57% of those who exercised regularly thought they did enough of it.

Normal growth and development in infancy should assure physical fitness for ordinary and even strenuous physical tasks because of innate, powerful drives toward functional development at this period of life. The infant who naturally strives for motor fitness can be on the way to a lifetime of improving physical fitness. The preschool child who characteristically uses his large muscles during many hours of the day is continuing a self-imposed program of physical fitness. Two- to 6-year-old children like to run, jump, climb, and balance themselves. They enjoy dancing, they are fond of rhythmic play, and they can use a cycle. They experiment in using their muscles in constantly growing fields of activity. As children approach elementary school age, their social development leads to increased activity in play with other children.

But, our present culture makes it difficult to maintain functional fitness. As children grow older, current sedentary life-styles tend to diminish opportunities for attaining physical fitness. Even preschool-age children use the many conveniences which eliminate physical effort.

Physical education should be a unique opportunity for increasing fitness with all children involved in tasks and activities which challenge their musculoskeletal and cardiopulmonary systems. If activities such as swimming, skiing, skating, cycling, hiking, running, and group competitive games are routinely enjoyed during childhood, there will be a tendency to continue such activities in later life. Inquiry, observation, and discussion about exercise and suitable ways to do it should lead parents to a better understanding of their children's needs. The pediatrician can be an important force by helping to form attitudes and influencing courses of action.

An estimate of physical fitness is an essential component of a health appraisal whether it is a periodic examination of a well child, a preschool or precamp evaluation, or an evaluation to authorize participation in strenuous exercise. It is

This statement has been reviewed and approved by the Academy's Council on Child Health.

312   Appendices

difficult to apply any of the recommended tests for evaluating fitness to infants and preschool children. However, the pediatrician can arrive at a reasonable estimate of fitness by specific questions about physical activity and by observing the child's strength, agility, coordination, and endurance throughout the interview and health examination. For example, asking if the infant pulls up to a standing position is routine in evaluating development. This activity also requires strength; and, if the question includes the length of time the infant can stand, endurance can be determined. Most pediatricians routinely ask if a young child can operate a tricycle or bicycle. But, also ask if he/she actually *does* it, *how often*, and for *how long.* "Can he/she swim?" could be followed by, "How often?" Also ask, "How long does he/she play during waking hours?" Questions about fatigue, response to exercise, and motivation for strenuous activity all rightfully belong in the health history.

Pediatricians have an important and obligatory role in advising and motivating parents about fitness aspects of the young child's development. The health benefits and the satisfactions from exercise, strenuous activity, and attainment of physical fitness may be established early in life by encouraging attitudes and behavior which carry over into later childhood and adult life. Thus, getting places "on your own," using stairways instead of elevators, and physical play instead of sedentary recreation may lead to activities later which have beneficial effects on preventing obesity, lowering the incidence of coronary heart disease and atherosclerosis, and increasing cardiopulmonary efficiency as well as developing a *joie de vivre.*

COMMITTEE ON PEDIATRIC ASPECTS OF PHYSICAL FITNESS, RECREATION, AND SPORTS
MELVIN L. THORNTON, M.D., *Chairman*
GLORIA D. ENG, M.D.
THOMAS G. FLYNN, M.D.
JOHN H. KENNELL, M.D.
ROBERT N. MCLEOD, JR., M.D.
THOMAS E. SHAFFER, M.D.
WILLIAM B. STRONG, M.D.
JOHN C. TOWER, M.D.
Consultant
NATHAN J. SMITH, M.D.
Liaison Representatives
JACK BELL, AMA Committee on Medical Aspects of Sports
LUCILLE BURKETT, National Association for Sport and Physical Education, AAHPER

BIBLIOGRAPHY
AAHPER Youth Fitness Test Manual, rev ed. Washington DC: American Alliance for Health, Physical Education, and Recreation, 1975.
Bailey DA: Exercise, fitness and physical education for the growing child—A concern. Can J Public Health 64:421, 1973.
Boyer JM: Effects of Chronic Exercise on Cardiovascular Function, Physical Fitness Research Digest. President's Council on Physical Fitness and Sports, series 2, No. 3, July 1972.
Clarke HH: Physical and Motor Tests in the Medford Boys' Growth Study. Englewood Cliffs, New Jersey, Prentice-Hall Inc, 1971.
National Adult Physical Fitness Survey: Newsletter (special ed), President's Council on Physical Fitness and Sports.
Johnson WR, Buskirk ER (eds): Science and Medicine of Exercise and Sports, ed 2. New York, Harper & Row, 1974.

JOINT COMMITTEE ON PHYSICAL FITNESS,
RECREATION, AND SPORTS MEDICINE

ATHLETIC ACTIVITIES BY CHILDREN WITH
SKELETAL ABNORMALITIES (RE0009)

A PHYSICIAN's recommendations concerning athletic activity for normal, healthy children must take into account a wide range of individual differences in size, age, coordination, stage of maturation, and level of physical and mental development. However, when the child has a skeletal abnormality, the physician must also consider the broad spectrum of variations of the disorder itself. For example, a child with rheumatoid arthritis may be in acute pain with systemic symptoms, may have no evidence of activity, may have mild monarticular arthritis that terminates after two or three years, or may have every joint involved without let-up for ten years.

The following principles will serve as a guide to the physician as he discusses athletic competition with the child and his parents.

It is important to distinguish between *participation in athletic activities* and *participation in competitive sports*. Competition is often highly motivating and may be a means for promoting self-satisfaction and developing muscles and coordination. But, this is so only *if the child is successful* in his competitive efforts. If a child is condemned to constant failure because of limitations in strength, endurance, range of motion, coordination, or for any cause, participation in competitive activities can be destructive to his self-image. A child with limited ability should be guided to an appropriate level of activities with no competition or with a goal of competition against one's previous performance. A child with a serious handicap usually recognizes that he has no opportunity to succeed; however, the child with a mild handicap which keeps him from ever being first or causes him always to come in last may experience considerable frustration and discouragement.

A child should be allowed to participate in formal and informal athletic activities with children of his own age, according to his abilities and interests. Any action that keeps a child from full participation with his peers should be considered carefully because it may affect his physical, social, and emotional development and may decrease his self-esteem and self-confidence. If restrictions are necessary, the reasons should be explained as clearly and reassuringly as possible. The duration of the restriction should be spelled out whenever possible, and substitute activities should be proposed to keep the child involved with his peers in group activities which offer some competition, excitement, or potential for muscle building or development of coordination. Several studies have shown that some parents of children with chronic disorders have a tendency to introduce restrictions or continue them contrary to the advice or intention of the physician. Studies have also shown that patients and their parents may misunderstand the physician's reasons for recommending restrictions and may have unwarranted concerns about the patient's health.

Other parents push their children into activities because of their own, rather than the child's, desire. A discussion with the parents and child should be arranged to find out who wants the youngster to participate in what activity, and why. With this information, a discussion with the physical education director, and a careful clinical evaluation of the child, the physician can counsel the parents and the child about the problems associated with the physical activity of a person with his handicap.

The physician should (1) keep restrictions to a minimum and remove them as soon as possible; (2) explain the reasons for the restrictions clearly and repeatedly; and (3) keep a child with a skeletal abnormal-

ATHLETICS AND SKELETAL ABNORMALITIES

ity in some physical activities with his peers, whenever possible.

The members of the Committee on Sports Medicine of the American Academy of Orthopaedic Surgeons were asked for recommendations about the following athletic competition for children with common skeletal abnormalities: (1) mild athletic competition: walking, bicycle riding, jogging; (2) moderate athletic competition: tennis, roller skating, ice skating, baseball, volley ball, swimming; and (3) vigorous athletic competition: football, skiing, soccer.

The orthopedic surgeons believe that no decisions are cut and dried, that x-rays or a history alone are usually not sufficient, that clinical findings should be correlated with x-rays, and that recommendations be individualized.

Activities for some conditions are:

1. Osgood-Schlatter's disease: Boys should be allowed to participate in vigorous athletic competition up to their pain tolerance. If the condition is acute, this generally means mild or no competition; if the condition is chronic, mild or moderate activity is advised.

2. Spondylolisthesis: If the condition is asymptomatic, moderate or vigorous athletic competition usually can be permitted. If a child with spondylolisthesis is symptomatic, he should be treated—usually with a back support and corrective exercises. If treatment renders him asymptomatic, he may be allowed to play basketball or football while wearing the back support. Basketball is more stressful for a patient with spondylolisthesis than football, and the twisting motion of baseball may incapacitate him.

3. Patients with a history of congenital subluxation of the hip, Legg-Perthes disease, slipped capital femoral epiphysis: In general, the recommendations for children who have had these conditions are the same: with mild deformity of the femoral head, moderate to vigorous, preferably noncontact, athletic competition; with moderate deformity, mild to moderate competi-

tion; and with severe deformity, mild or no competition. However, the compensation by the acetabulum and the amount of motion in the hip are other important considerations. Clinically, if there is mild limitation of motion in the hip, the joint space is good, and muscle function about the hip is strong, the child should be able to compete through the high school level without difficulty. However, if there is moderate limitation of motion in the hip, the child is not a candidate for collision sports such as football and wrestling, and probably not a candidate for basketball. If he is too active, recurring hip pain will develop with too much frequency, and restriction to a level where there is no hip pain and no spasms will be required. Swimming and nonweight bearing activities will be tolerated by all children with these conditions.

4. Recommendations for athletic competition for a child on steroid therapy when the underlying disease (for example, asthma) is not active and not a factor in the decision: during long-term, low dose or intermittent steroids, moderate or vigorous activity; immediately following a two- to four-week course of steroids with cushinoid changes, mild to moderate activity; six months to one year after cessation of steroid therapy, vigorous activity.

5. A child with rheumatoid arthritis: disease quiescent with complete functional recovery, moderate to vigorous activity; disease quiescent with minimal or moderate crippling, mild to moderate activity (especially ice skating or swimming); complete functional recovery but still on full salicylate therapy, mild to moderate activity; asymptomatic with mild effusion and synovial changes in weight-bearing joints and on full salicylate therapy, mild activity with participation at own level of tolerance.

JOINT COMMITTEE ON PHYSICAL FITNESS,
   RECREATION, AND SPORTS MEDICINE
EUGENE F. DIAMOND, M.D., *Chairman*
JOHN C. HEFFELFINGER, M.D., Committee on Accident Prevention
JOHN KENNELL, M.D., Committee on Children with Handicaps

AMERICAN ACADEMY OF PEDIATRICS

JOHN R. PONCHER, M.D., Committee on
School Health, 1971-1972
E. C. SHACKLEFORD, JR., M.D., Committee on School Health
THOMAS E. SHAFFER, M.D., Committee

on Youth
MELVIN L. THORNTON, M.D., AMA
Committee on the Medical Aspects
of Sports

Sports Medicine

Numbers in bold face indicate a figure or table.

A

AAHPERD Health-Related Fitness Test, 127
Abduction stress test for medial collateral ligament, **234**
Acclimatization, insufficient, as cause of heat-related illness, 90
Acetaminophen, 215
Achilles tendinitis, 177-78
Acne, 112
Adductor test, 231
Adenosine triphosphate (ATP), 117
Adipose tissue, 101
Adiposity, 120
Adolescents
    aortic stenosis in, 254
    diets of, 102
    maturation of, 33-34, **58, 59**
    multiple dystrophy in, 255
    scoliosis in, 255
    suggested physical activities for, 20-21
Aerobic conditioning, 126
    and changes in muscle metabolism, 126
    and changes in the cardiovascular system, 125
    and changes in ventilation, 125
Aerobic exercise, 20
Aerobic fitness, increasing, 122-23
Aerobic function and performance, of female athlete, 36-37
Aerobic metabolism, **132**
Aerobic power
    determining, 121
    relative contributions of, **133**
Aerobic value, of selected sports, **28**
Aerobic work, 117
Age appropriateness, and team sports, 21

Aircast, 212
Albuterol, 252
Alopecia, 112
Amenorrhea, 40-41, 103
    primary, 40
    secondary, 40
American Alliance for Health, Physical Education, Recreation, and Dance (AAHPERD), 127
American Coaching Effectiveness Program, 23
Amnesia, 236
    anterograde, 237
    retrograde, 236-37
Anabolic steroids. See Steroids
Anaerobic capacity, 119
Anaerobic conditioning, 123-24
Anaerobic exercise, role of carbohydrates in, 100
Anaerobic metabolism, **132**
Anaerobic power, relative contributions of, **133**
Anaerobic training, 126
Analgesics, in management of soft-tissue trauma, 214, **219**
Anemia
    iron-deficiency, 49, 102, 103
    runner's, 103
Ankle sprain
    classification of, 198
    cryotherapy for, **217-18**
    inflatable splint for, **217**
    rehabilitation of, 198-201
Anomalous left coronary artery, 75
Anorexia nervosa, 90
Anterior cruciate ligament, 232
Anterior leg pain syndrome, 179
Anterograde amnesia, 237
Anti-inflammatory drugs, 175-176
    nonsteroidal, **187**, 215
Aortic stenosis (AS), 254-55
Apophysitis of
    posterior calcaneus (Sever Disease), 176
    tibial tubercle, 178

D

Dehydration
  inadvertent, 88
  prevention of, 88
Delayed menarche, 39
Diabetes insipidus, 90
Diabetes mellitus, 90, 254, **258**
Diaphyseal (greenstick) fracture,
    225-26
Diet. *See also* Athletic diet
  and cystic fibrosis, 253
  and diabetes mellitus, 254
Dimethyl sulfoxide (DMSO), 176
Disabled child, participation of, in
    sports activities, 21-22
Disease status, associated, as
    cause of overuse
    syndrome, 174
Dislocations, 227. *See also*
    Fractures
  cervical, 243
  of the patella, 232-33
Drawer test for anterior and
    posterior movement,
    234
Drug testing of athletes, 112-13
Dysmenorrhea, 44
Dysrhythmia, 255

E

Edema, 214
Electrocardiogram, 76
Elevation, in management of soft-
    tissue trauma, 214, **219**
Endurance training, 101
Environment, improper, as cause
    of overuse syndrome,
    173
Epicondylitis of the humerus, 33
Epidural hematoma, 238
Epilepsy, 256
Epiphyseal injuries, Salter-Harris
    classification, **229**
Epiphyseal/physeal fracture,
    223-24
Epiphysis progressive
    maturation, **229**
Epiphysitis of the medial
    epicondyle, 182-83
Equipment
  appropriate and injury
    prevention, 162

improper, as cause of
    overuse syndrome,
    173-74
Estrogen, 38
  deficiency in, 40-41, 103
Eumenorrhea, 40
Exercise
  in cold environment, 92-93
  duration of, and aerobic
    fitness, 122
  effect of, on expiratory flow
    rate, **259**
  frequency of, and aerobic
    fitness, 122
  impact of heat on, 84-85
  intensity of, and aerobic
    fitness, 122
  type of, and aerobic fitness,
    123
Exercise-induced asthma (EIA),
    251

F

Fat. *See also* Body fat
  role of, in athletic diet, 101
Female athlete(s), 36
  aerobic function and
    performance of, 36-37
  body composition of, 36
  breasts of, 44
  gynecologic considerations
    of, 38
    amenorrhea in, 40-41,
      103
    contraceptives, 43
    delayed menarche, 39
    dysmenorrhea in, 44
    eumenorrhea in, 40
    infertility, 43
    irregular menses, 40
    menses, 38-39, 40
    menstrual dysfunction,
      39-40, 41
    menstrual physiology,
      38
    and negative proges-
      terone challenge
      test, 42
    osteoporosis and
      amenorrheic
      athletes, 42-43

324

Physical education class,
excusing child from, 23,
252-253, 254, 256
Physical examination record,
73-74
Physical fitness, 117
body composition, 120
factors influencing, 121
anaerobic conditioning,
123-24
conditioning, 121
duration of exercise, 122
frequency of exercise,
122
habitual activity, 124-25
increasing flexibility, 123
intensity of exercise, 122
specificity of training,
121
type of exercise, 123
flexibility, 120
responses to exercise,
117-18
cardiovascular, 118
increasing workloads,
118
oxygen consump-
tion (VO$_2$max),
119
muscle metabolic, 119
ventilatory, 119
Physical Therapy Practice Act,
208
Physician. See also Team
physician
fitness testing in office of,
127-28
need for, at stations
examination, 50, 51
role of, in providing guidance
on physical activity, 18
Physiologic effects
of conditioning, **131**
of exercise in the heat, 84-85
Plantar fasciitis, 177
Postconcussion syndrome, 237
Posttraumatic migraine, 238
Pre-event meals, 104-5
Premature ventricular
contractions (PVC), 77
Premenstrual syndrome (PMS),
43

Preparticipation evaluation,
duties of team physician
in, 189
Preschoolers. See Toddlers and
preschoolers
Preseason conditioning, 161
President's Council on Physical
Fitness and Sports, 126
Priapism, 112
Primary amenorrhea, 40
Progesterone challenge test
negative, 42
positive, 42
Progressive resistance exercises,
200
Protective equipment, safety
rules regarding, 20
Protein, in athletic diet, 101-2
Pseudoanemia, 102-3
Pubertal development
of female pubic hair, **59**
of male pubic hair, **58**
Puncture wound, 220-21

Q

Quadriplegia, 161
transient, 244

R

Radiographs for neck injuries,
246
Range-of-motion (ROM)
exercises, 199
Reconditioning, 176
Rehabilitation, 196-97
guidelines for, 197-98
phase I: acute injury,
199, **204**
phase II: initial rehabilitation, 199-200, **204**
phase III: progressive
rehabilitation,
200-201, **204**
phase IV: integrated
functions, 201, **205**
phase V: return to sport,
201, **205**
inflammation/pain/
performance cycle, **206**
injury and inflammation in,
197

principles of, 196
role of athletic trainer in,
209-10
sprains and strains
guidelines, **203**
Respiratory illnesses
bronchial asthma, 251-52
cystic fibrosis, 252-53
Rest, in management of soft-
tissue trauma, 212
Rest, ice, compression, and
elevation (RICE), 199,
212-14
Retrograde amnesia, 236-37
Rheumatic fever, 215
Roentgenogram, 76
"Roid rage," 112
Rule changes, and injury
prevention, 162
Runner's anemia, 103

S

Salter-Harris Classification in
epiphyseal injuries, **229**
Salt tablets, use of, 89-90
School-aged children
maturation of, 32-33
suggested physical activity
for, 19-20
Scoliosis, 255
Secondary amenorrhea, 40
Second impact syndrome, 240
Sever disease, 176
Shin splints (anterior leg pain
syndrome), 179
Shoulder impingement
syndromes, 181-82
Skiing, sports injuries in, 155-57,
170
Skin fold caliper, 137
measurement error using,
138
use of, 138-39
Slow acclimatization to heat, 86
Soccer, sports injuries in, 154-55,
170
Soft-tissue trauma
initial management of, 212
analgesics in, 214-15
compression in, 214,
219
elevation in, 214

ice (cryotherapy),
213-14
rest in, 212
treatment of sprained
ligament, **219**
Spearing, 241, 242
Special Olympics, 256
Specificity of training, influence
of, on fitness, 121-22
Spineboard, 245
Spironolactone, 43
Splenic rupture, 52
Spondylolysis, 151, 159
Spondylolysis/Spondylolisthesis,
183-84
Sports
and academics, 22
aerobic value of selected, **28**
and co-ed participation in, 22
disabled participation in,
21-22
effects of, on fitness
components, **129-30**
stress in, 22-23
Sports anemia, 102
Sports facilities, 188
Sports injuries, 22, **169**. See also
Overuse syndromes
in baseball, 148-50, **169**
in basketball, 152, **169**
epidemiologic studies in,
146-48
factors in prevention of, **171**
football, 150-52, **169**
in gymnastics, 158-59, **170**
of head. See Head injuries
in hockey, **170**
in ice hockey, 159-61
of knee. See Knee injuries
of neck. See Neck injuries
prevention of, 161-63
prevention of in neck, 247
skiing, 155-57, **170**
soccer, 154-55, **170**
in track, 157-58
in wrestling, 152-54, **170**
Sports medicine program,
responsibilities of
athletic trainer in, 210
Sports participation health
record, **55-57**
Sports preparticipation
examination, 48
examination, 50